Acta Neurochirurgica
Supplements

Editor: H.-J. Reulen
Assistant Editor: H.-J. Steiger

# Neurosurgery and Medical Ethics

## Edited by
## H. August van Alphen

## Acta Neurochirurgica
## Supplements 74

Springer-Verlag Wien GmbH

H. August van Alphen, M.D., Ph.D.
Department of Neurosurgery, Academisch Ziekenhuis Vrije Universiteit,
Amsterdam, The Netherlands

© 1999 Springer-Verlag Wien

Softcover reprint of the hardcover 1st edition 1999

Typesetting: Asco Trade Typesetting Ltd., Hong Kong


Graphic design: Ecke Bonk
Printed on acid-free and chlorine free bleached paper
SPIN: 10730592

With 1 Figure

**Library of Congress Cataloging-in-Publication Data**

Neurosurgery and medical ethics / edited by H. August van Alphen.
    p.    cm. – (Acta neurochirurgica.    Supplement,    ISSN 0065-1419
; 74)
    Includes bibliographical references and index.
    ISBN 978-3-7091-7310-7     ISBN 978-3-7091-6387-0 (eBook)
    DOI 10.1007/978-3-7091-6387-0
    1. Nervous system–Surgery–Moral and ethical aspects Congresses.
2. Medical ethics Congresses. I. Alphen, H. A. M. van.
II. Series.
    [DNLM: 1. Neurosurgery Congresses. 2. Ethics, Medical Congresses.
W1 AC8661 no. 74 1999]
RD593.N418 1999
617.4'8–dc21
DNLM/DLC
for Library of Congress                                                          99-33462
                                                                                 CIP


ISSN 0065-1419

# Preface

This supplement of Acta Neurochirurgica contains the proceedings of the Ninth Convention of the Academia Eurasiana Neurochirurgica held in Château St. Gerlach, Houthem, The Netherlands, 29 July – 1 August 1998. During this convention a three-day symposium on Neurosurgery and Medical Ethics was held.

In this time of tremendous technical advancement in medicine in general and neurosurgery in particular, we are liable to lose sight of the sick patient as a human being, and the odds are that he will be the object rather than the subject of our action in the near future. It is a purpose and a task of the Academia Eurasiana Neurochirurgica to recognize this thread and to pay attention to tradition, morality and ethics in neurological surgery. The theme of this convention and the subject of the symposium met this purpose as no other.

In the scientific sessions during the first day, the moral backgrounds of medical ethics in the most important cultures and religions in east and west were elucidated by invited experts in this field. A mutual respectful understanding of each other's conception of and belief in ethical principles is a growing necessity in our multicultural societies in both continents. On the second day, the ethical aspects of different fields of neurological surgery were discussed by members of the Academia. In this context, also the internationally much-discussed and much-criticized regulations on euthanasia in The Netherlands were explained. During the last morning, there were some papers and ample discussions on: How to educate our pupils in moral attitude and ethical behaviour?

The convention was a very successful and highly inspiring gathering. We wish to express our sincere thanks to all speakers and participants for their contribution. We felt, that these contributions would be well worth reading for all physicians and others, working in different fields of medicine. It was a great pleasure, indeed, to edit this book for this purpose. I also like to cordially thank Ms. Susanne Mayr of the Production Department of Springer, Wien New York for her generous dedication and great help in realizing this issue.

Amsterdam, July 1999

*H. August van Alphen, M.D., Ph.D.*
*Past President A.E.A.N., Editor*

# Contents

**Opening Ceremony**
**Ninth Convention of the Academia Eurasiana Neurochirurgica**

Acta Neurochir (1999) [Suppl] 74: 3–4

# Presidential Welcome Address

## H. August van Alphen

Department of Neurosurgery, Academisch Ziekenhuis Vrije Universiteit, Amsterdam, The Netherlands

## Dear Academicians, Dear Guests, Ladies and Gentlemen.

It is my great pleasure and honour, indeed, to cordially welcome you all to this 9th convention of the Academia Eurasiana Neurochirurgica. After having had the meetings in Seoul, Copenhagen and Sydney as from 1992, we are very proud to serve as the Academy's host in Europe this time, and to have you with us in this wonderful ambiance of Château St. Gerlach in this most beautiful part of the Netherlands.

The original designation of "Academia" referred to the grove in which Plato's school of philosophy in ancient Greece took place and hence to the philosophical ambiance itself. The academies, founded in Europe from the fifteenth century onwards, were philosophical clubs or communities of like-minded men, devoting themselves to the pursuit of learning in an atmosphere of friendship, leisure, and ease, preferably in a country house far from the towns.

So, it is obvious that through the years the venue of the academies always played a prominent role in their gatherings. That is, why we searched all over the country to find an appropriate location for this meeting of the Academia Eurasiana Neurochirurgica. And I think, we succeeded in our aim quite well.

An appropriate venue will also facilitate the second criterion of the concept of "Academia", which is: to meet as a congenial group of people, who want to have discussions in an atmosphere of friendship, leisure and ease, and in this way, as is written in the constitution of our academy, to promote scientific, academic, social and cultural exchanges and mutual understanding between neurosurgeons of Asia and Europe. All of you, who attended earlier conventions, know, that this principle is very much alive in this Academia. I really

hope, that this convention may further intensify this solidarity and friendship.

But the real reason and aim to gather with this academy is to discuss and to philosophise on serious matters, and again according to the constitution, to strengthen the traditions and ethics of neurological surgery.

The theme and subject of the present scientific meeting: Neurosurgery and Medical Ethics, perfectly fits this purpose of the Academia Eurasiana Neurochirurgica.

Medical practice, and specifically neurosurgical practice, is becoming more and more complex. The technical developments during the last decades, both in diagnostic and in therapeutic respects, are immense and facinating and have brought blessing and happiness to many patients. But almost daily, we also experience, that these growing technical opportunities more and more touch moral boundaries and may cause great ethical problems.

These moral boundaries, however, are not the same for everybody, not even in the same country or in the same hospital, let alone in different countries or different continents. It is not our intention and it will be even impossible to draw up a set of ethical rules for neurological surgery or to aim for a mondial consensus on ethical standards in neurosurgery during this meeting. But in this multicultural society, it at least is necessary to be informed of the different views of medical ethics in different cultures and religions for a good mutual understanding and respect.

We thought that the Academia meeting would be the ideal setting for exploration, discussion and reflection on the different opinions in this field in Asia and Europe. During this symposium we will hear about the moral backgrounds of medical ethics from the perspective of the most important cultures and religions of these continents. We will discuss the ethical aspects of different fields of neurosurgical practice. And we will try to find out how we can teach our pupils moral attitude and ethical behaviour in the best way.

At the same time, our ladies will have the opportunity to explore and reflect on the beauty and the treasure of this wonderful estate, the Limburg landscape and city of Maastricht. And for real leisure, a special programme has been designed, which will let you taste of the culture, tradition and the culinary delights of this area of The Netherlands.

Dear friends, welcome to Houthem–St. Gerlach, welcome to this Convention of the Academia Eurasiana Neurochirurgica. I really hope, you will meet wisdom and friendship and will enjoy your stay with us during these days.

Correspondence: H. August van Alphen, M.D., Ph.D., Hogerlustlaan 57, 1191 CL Ouderkerk a/d Amstel, The Netherlands.

Acta Neurochir (1999) [Suppl] 74: 5–6

# Opening Address to the 9th Convention

**K. Sano**

Fuji Brain Institute & Hospital, Fujinomiya, Japan

## Academicians! Distinguished Guests! Ladies and Gentlemen!

President, Prof. van Alphen asked me to give some thoughts on the meaning and importance of a scientific academy in general and the Academia Eurasiana Neurochirurgica in particular. I feel greatly honoured to accept his invitation. As you know, the Greek "Academeia" (ἀκαδήμεια), academia in Latin, was said to derive its name from a mythological hero, Hekademos or Academus (Ἀκάδημος) who, according to legend, revealed to Castor and Pollux, where Theseus had hidden the young Helen with whom Theseus had eloped, so that the Dioscuri could bring back Helen who later became the famous beauty of the Trojan War. Academia was the name of a shrine and an olive grove located about one mile north-west of the city wall of ancient Athens. The area was improved and adorned by Cimon (510–449 B.C.), an Athenian statesman and a general and a hero of the Battle of Salamis.

He bequeathed the property to his fellow citizens as a public park. This Academy was the favourite resort of Plato (428–348 B.C.) (Πλάτων) and here he taught for nearly 50 years. From the name of the Park his school received the name of Academic. Rome had no academies but Cicero (106–43 B.C.) termed his villa "Academia" and here composed his "Academic Questions".

The word later became associated with certain forms of educational institutions and appeared in English in the 15th century. It was adopted by many learned groups to indicate an association of people engaged in the same scientific, professional or cultural pursuits. Shakespeare used the word "academe" instead of academy. In his "Love's Labour's Lost",

Ferdinand, King of Navarre said, "Our court shall be a little Academe (I i 13). And Biron, a noble man maintained,

"From women's eyes this doctrine I derive:
They sparkle still the right Promethean fire;
They are the books, the arts, the academes,
That show, contain and nourish all the world:
Else none at all in aught proves excellent (IV iii 347–351)."

The most famous academy is l'Académie Française, which was established by Cardinal de Richelieu (1585–1642) in 1634 and incorporated in 1635, existing, except for an interruption during the era of the French Revolution, to the present day. The first scientific academies were begun in the 16th century, with the founding of the Academia Secretorum Naturae by an Italian philosopher and scientist Giambattista della Porta in 1560. The English Royal Society and the French Académie des Sciences began as informal gatherings of famous men. The "Invisible College" of London and Oxford, which had its first meetings in 1645, was incorporated as the Royal Society in 1662. In Paris a group including Descartes and Pascal started private meetings almost at the same time. In 1699 the society was established at the Louvre under the name of Académie des Sciences. In the 18th century the fame and achievements of the Royal Society and of the Académie des Sciences were internationally recognized, and many European countries started to found their own national academy of sciences.

The American Academy of Neurological Surgery which was founded in 1938, has slightly different authority as compared with these European academies. It, however, stimulated Hans Werner Pia and myself, who were at that time honorary members of the Academy, to dream of founding the Eurasian Academy of Neurosurgery. Prof. Pia and I consulted many friends about this matter in 1983 and 1984, and were helped by Prof. Jean Brihaye and Prof. Emil Pasztor, to name only a few. When we had to create the logo of the Academia, Prof. Pia asked me to coin the motto which should be put into the logo. I replied, "Humanitate et Arte" (with humanity and art). Prof. Pia changed it to "Humanitati et Arti" (to humanity and to art). He meant by this, the Academia is dedicated to Humanity and to Art, both of which are equally the backbone and the symbol of the Academia. Finally, in 1985, our first Convention was held in Bonn, Bundesrepublik Deutschland under the presidency of Prof. Pia.

Unfortunately, on the 9th of July in 1986, Prof. Pia passed away to our great sorrow. In the same year, from October the 5th to the 8th, the second Convention was orgnized by myself in Hakone, Japan, and in the following year Prof. Brihaye held the 3rd Convention in Brussels. The Academy's charter specifies that the purposes of the organization are not only to pro-

mote scientific-academic exchange and mutual understanding between neurosurgeons of Europe and Asia but to strengthen the tradition and ethics of neurological surgery and also to broaden neurosurgeons' world views based on the humanities. The subject of this 9th Convention meets these purposes very well.

*As Goethe wrote:*

"Wir sind naturforschend Pantheisten, dichtend Polytheisten, sittlich Monotheisten. (Maximen und Reflexionen 807)" (We are pantheists as natural scientists, polytheists as poets, and morally monotheists.) We, as medical "Naturforscher", always feel the divine existence when we see and treat patients and follow the course of their diseases. That is the basis of our medical ethics. We look forward to listening to presentations and expression of thoughts of the participants.

Correspondence: Keiji Sano, M.D., Ph.D., Fuji Brain Institute & Hospital, 270-12 Sugita, Fujinomiya 4180021 Japan.

Acta Neurochir (1999) [Suppl] 74: 7–9

# The Twain have met!

## A. Hoytink

Director-General for Asia and the Pacific of the Dutch Ministry of Foreign Affairs, The Netherlands

Your organizing committee has been courageous enough to give me the honour of delivering an opening address at this learned gathering, since I have neither an ethical nor a neurosurgical background. It is nevertheless my intention to point out some differences in conceptions of Asian and European mentalities which should of course lead to divergent bio-ethical philosophies and practices. I base myself on my experiences over more than 14 years in Asia. I hope to have you share with me the final result of our mental tour of Asia and Europe, which will be that significant differences do exist, but that in fact they do matter less and less for the subject matter of this introduction.

## First of all: Asia and Europe

When the average European thinks of Asia, he visualizes just one huge part of the world. Not everybody is aware that Asia is so multi-facetted. As for religions there are monotheists, pantheists, philosophers like the Buddhists (of whom there are several "branches") and animists. There is Southeast Asia, Nepal and Sri Lanka with their Buddhism; there is huge India with its hundreds of millions of Hindus; Pakistan, Malaysia, Indonesia, Iran, Afghanistan with their great number of muslims, sometimes subdivided into Shiites and others. There is the only almost fully Roman Catholic nation in the region, the Philippines. There is also that combination of philosophy, tradition and some beliefs in a creator, which leads to Shintoism, Confucianism and the teachings of Lao Tse in Japan, Korea and China. Their attitudes with regard to the medical practice and its ethics were likely to be as divergent as their theological ideas. And yet, through contacts with Europe, the medical profession began to mutually influence one another. Chinese medical methods and medicines reached Europe hundreds of years ago. Japanese scientists learned Dutch in order to be able to read medical treatises in the original. By the way, the first international treaty, whereby the Americans opened Japan to the world in the 1850's had to be written in Dutch, the only European language they know, just as a result of the Japanese ability to read the Dutch medical books.

My knowledge of the details of ethical standards of the different Asia's is explicably almost non-existent. But judging from the high standards of civilization and the moral influence of their religions, which all have a high ethical component, (for instance the Buddhist respect for live, the Chinese family values) I feel justified in assuming that basically they were shared by us all. Many Europeans, specially the Christians, were influenced by the teachings of the great medieval philospher Thomas Aquinas. He stated that all men are subjects of and guided by the "law of nature". Through this innate law our behaviour, especially in its social and moral context, is always regulated by supernatural laws. I am convinced that he did not mean that for only Europeans but for all mankind.

Around the middle of the 19th century medical practice and medical knowledge burgeoned into an explosive development. Thanks to modern communications, the learning of foreign languages, the exchange of learned reseachers, the medical world has becomes a "global village" and shares their experiences. Together, Asians, Europeans and Americans, are improving, inventing and applying their discoveries which, in most cases, lead to publications, so that every member of the profession might make use of it or is warned of thus far unknown hasards. Worldwide, people now wrestle with existential questions, implying the value of life. To mention but a few, the choice for or against abortion and euthanasia, the "in vitro fertilization" and the dilemma about embryonal residuals. There also is the question whether embryonal matter may be used for research to find an answer to, for example, Parkinson's disease; the question of birth planning by artificial means, specially in the context of poverty or overpopulation, the transplantation of organs and the control of how these organs were obtained (the difference between an organ being given or just taken away without the informed consent of the donor).

There are many more moral and ethical problems of course. However, thanks to good communication these days, which I mentioned before, the dilemmas are clear and solutions are being studied. The WHO in its declerations of Geneva and, among others, of Tokyo, is progressing in reaching and formulating ever more guidelines for the direction of the consciences of all concerned in the medical profession.

Although medical practice has always been the subject of ethical critique, two recent developments in particular have served to transform the traditional notion of medical ethics: (1) advances in medicine and health care due to the influence of biotechnology and technology-oriented medicine, and (2) the rapidly changing socio-cultural context marked by the prevalence of a plurality of values in western countries, especially those values which bear on the provision of health care.

The socio-cultural context of medical practice has changed in many respects. During the last three decades, the influence of religious values in the resolution of moral problems in medicine has diminished whereas a nonreligiously, secularly-grounded normative view of human life has become more influential. This view emphasises personal autonomy and each patient's right to make his or her own health care decisions. At the same time, some philosophers focused on the power of health care professionals in present-day society, as well as on the socalled "medicalisation" of postmodern culture. Such critiques have resulted in a change in attitude toward health care professionals and an increasing demand by patients to participate in medical decisionmaking at virtually every level – not only in the physician-patient encounter but also within the health care system as such.

The social status of physicians has been affected significantly by these factors. Traditionally, 'medical ethics' referred to the deontology of the medical profession, to codes of conduct which consist partly of ordinary moral rules, partly of rules of etiquette, and partly of rules of professional conduct. In this sense bio-ethics has the following characteristics:

It is essentially a set of problems that focus on the internal morality of medicine, viz., those values, norms, and rules intrinsic to the actual practice of health care. Medicine is not considered a merely technical enterprise which can be morally evaluated from some exogenous standpoint. On the contrary, the professional practice of medicine always presumes and implies a moral perspective or point of view; therefore, what is judged to be sound medical practice is determined by the shared rules and standard procedures of the practice.

Since it was primarily concerned with explicating norms and formulating standards of professional conduct, medical ethics and etiquette have been segregated for a long time from general intellectual history. Moreover, before the 1960's, medical ethics was not a subject frequently discussed in public fora and the extant literature. Apparently, there was a consensus of opinion concerning the moral commitments of those who provided medical care, and the *explanation or codification* of these commitments was regarded as the principal concern of medical professionals.

A result of the gradual transformation of medical ethics is two-fold: First, it has produced a new professional – the health care ethicist or 'bio-ethicist' who possesses a specific body of knowledge and particular cognitive skills; who publishes in specialized journals, participates in newly-formed societies, and teaches in newly-established centers, institutes, and departments. Second, it has produced a new socio-cultural interest in medico-moral matters of significant public concern – particularly in those countries where advanced biomedical technology permeates public as well as private life. 'Bio-ethics' is a way of publicly addressing, explaining and debating problems generated by science and technology.

Today there is growing concern that the results of the aforesaid transformation are unsatisfactory. Professionalisation and institutionalisation of medical ethics received an enormous stimulus because both the adequacy and the relevance of medicine's internal morality were put into question.

Professional ethicists have placed more and more emphasis on the crucial role of external morality: the principles, norms, and rules operative in society which bear on medicine and are frequently codified in law. Thus, for some, medicine and health care are nothing more than interesting "intellectual" phenomena with respect to which general ethical theories, principles, and rules may be applied.

Through this historical process emphasis is placed on the common good, and this was combined with an appeal to the self-interest of the members of the profession. Social recognition could only be gained on the basis of a strong internal organization and self-imposed standards of behaviour. Self-regulation by physicians and a special style of life, structured in terms of high ideals, duties, and virtues, could promote the physician's image, and thus the power and prestige of each member of the medical profession.

This gathering, which starts today, could provide a strong impetus to the developments of bio-ethical concepts to guide us. Therefore I wish you all the wisdom to proceed in the path of finding further directions for which members of your distinguished and noble profession *must* be looking in the search for guidance for his "Asian–European" conscience.

Your Academy indeed is a very important "vehicle" on that path. May its activities be blessed with enlightment in the coming days.

Correspondence: Ad Hoytink, LL.M., Postweg 12, 6523 LC Nijmegen, The Netherlands.

Acta Neurochir (1999) [Suppl] 74: 11–12

# Welcome Address on Behalf of the Netherlands Society of Neurosurgeons

C. J. J. Avezaat

Department of Neurosurgery, Academisch Ziekenhuis Rotterdam, Rotterdam, The Netherlands

## Mr. President, Members of The Academia Eurasiana Neurochirurgica, Ladies and Gentlemen

It is a great pleasure for me, as President of the Netherlands Society of Neurosurgeons, to speak a word of welcome to you, participants of the Ninth Convention of The Eurasian Academy of Neurological Surgery.

Apart from what I read in the introduction by your president in the final announcement of this meeting, I am not very familiar with the roots of your academy. One might wonder, on what common grounds, ideals or aims neurosurgeons from two continents of the old world have united themselves in a separate society. The answer is, I guess, that you are gathered here not so much on the basis of what you have in common, your neurosurgical profession, as rather on the basis of your differences with regard to race, society, culture, religion and political background. As I am saying this, I feel some sort of relief in being able to emphasize the differences between people in stead of denying them or covering them up, as seems to be the trend nowadays.

Your differences will not affect your professional standards. The clipping of an aneurysm will, or at least should, not be different whether it be done by a catholic or a protestant, a white or a black man, a man or a woman. At the most, the means which are at your disposal will differ according to the economic situation in your countries. However, the final object of our medical practice is not the sickness but the sick person and this person has a race, gender, culture, religion of his own. Our duty to act in the interest of the patient goes beyond that of treating the disease. This adds another dimension to our medical practice, that of medical ethics which constitutes the difference between medicine as a science and medicine as an art.

What does it take to be ethical neurosurgeons? It requires reflection on our own moral values. Since, according to Collins [2], besides family and formal education, religious experience, culture and social groups are the most common donors of ethical behaviour, it seems most appropriate to discuss medical ethics at a meeting of this kind. Therefore, Mr. President, I ought to congratulate you on the topic which has been chosen for this meeting: Neurosurgery and Medical Ethics.

With regard to medical ethics, our country, The Netherlands, is often considered in the international scene as "the odd man out", a special case, and this in a rather negative sense. Our often highly praised liberal and tolerant national character is less appreciated as far as our attitude towards the abuse of drugs and continuation-of-life decisions is concerned. Recently, an important European head of state as well as the adviser of the American President on the control of drug-abuse have referred to the so-called bad situation on drugs in The Netherlands. Not long ago, our minister of foreign affairs and the minister of health visited the Vatican to explain our policy on euthanasia to representatives of the Roman Catholic church. In discussions with foreign colleagues on the subject of euthanasia, I am sometimes deeply afflicted when I notice that their judgment is based on ignorance or prejudice.

The actual situation on euthanasia in The Netherlands is that it is forbidden by law. However, under specific circumstances no legal proceedings will be instituted: a voluntary and persistent request by the patient, an incurable disease with unbearable mental or physical suffering which cannot be relieved by any other solution, and concurrence of a second, independent physician. Detailed records should be kept and a non-natural cause of death should be declared.

Personally, my main problem is how to reconcile one's own conviction with regard to the right of self-determination and to the meaning of life and suffering with one's duties as a physician to stand by the patient until the end of the road. In this respect, I appreciate very much the juridical notion of "force majeure" or "circumstances beyond one's control". In my view, this means that there is only one option left to act in the interest of the patient, whereas all other options mean "letting the patient down". In such a situation there should be, however strangely it may sound to some of you, a "good feeling". Without this feeling there can be no euthanasia.

On the other hand, I can see that western society is still moving away from the statement by Callahan [1] [1] that "death is a part of life, to be accepted, and the grief that goes with it, to be endured". In this respect, I believe, we can learn from our fellow men from the east and from the south. As a young doctor, I worked for three years in a rural hospital in Bukumbi, near Mwanza, at the shores of Lake Victoria in Tanzania. Sometimes, when I made my rounds through the wards, it appeared that a patient, who had been critically ill the day before and was surely going to die, had disappeared. I then asked the nurse in Kiswahili "Mgonjwa, amekwenda wapi?". (The patient, where did he go?). And the nurse, slightly embarrassed, looking aside, invariably answered: "Mganga, doctor, his relatives came during the night and took him home to die". The fact that they came during the night in order not to have to pay the hospital bill was well taken by us.

Mr. President, ladies and gentlemen, sensing the atmosphere of this place and in this church, it is my impression that the organisers of this meeting have created the right ambiance for a frank and open exchange of ideas on these difficult issues. On behalf of our neurosurgical society, I wish you a good meeting and a pleasant stay in this beautiful part of our country.

Thank you

## References

1. Callahan D (1993) The troubled dream of life. Living with mortality. Simon & Schuster, New York
2. Collins WF (1995) Ethics and etiquette in neurosurgery. In: Award IA (ed) Philosophy of neurological surgery. Park Ridge, Illinois. Am Ass Neuro Surg, pp 41–48
3. Kaufman HH (1995) The Philosophy of dying and death. In: Award IHA (ed) Philosophy of neurological surgery. Park Ridge, Illinois. Am Ass Neurol Surg, pp 79–103

Correspondence: Cees J. J. Avezaat, M.D., Ph.D., Department of Neurosurgery, Academisch Ziekenhuis Rotterdam, Dr. Molewaterplein 40, 3015 GD Rotterdam, The Netherlands.

# Symposium Neurosurgery and Medical Ethics

Acta Neurochir (1999) [Suppl] 74: 15–16

# Introduction

## H. August van Alphen

Department of Neurosurgery, Academisch Ziekenhuis Vrije Universiteit, Amsterdam, The Netherlands

In his graduation address to the medical students of Jefferson Medical College, Philadelphia in 1926 – an address which he entitled "Consecratio Medici" – Harvey Cushing delineated the ethical standard in medicine in his time; he called this "common devotion". He defined common devotion in the following way: "Devotion is an attribute one cannot estimate and record by ordinary standards. How much the practising doctor cares about his patients as individuals apart from their being the source of his livelihood; how much the medical scientist may be interested in promoting science rather than in securing his own promotion; how much the teacher influences his pupils to their best efforts, unmindful of what the curriculum briefly requires of him; how much the student engages in his work for the work's sake, regardless of his marks and rating – all these things depend on a devotion which places spiritual above material rewards" [1]. With this statement, Cushing criticized the debasement of clinical practice, the overemphasis on research and the search for personal gain amongst his colleagues. He considered these to be the most important moral hazards in medicine at that time. This moral standard, defined by Cushing some 70 years ago, sounds very modern, even today, and by and large, is still valid. Numerous new developments in the last decades have, however, made medical practice far more complex than it was in Cushing's time, and have added many ethical problems and hazards to those mentioned above.

The technical boom in medicine, both in diagnostic and in therapeutic respects, has brought blessing and happiness to many patients. But these growing medical opportunities also constitute the hazard of people refusing to accept certain physical or mental shortcoming or defects any longer. They also constitute the trend of measuring the value of human life in medical or even economical criteria, instead of considering human life as being something unique itself.

The auspicious and favourable technical advances in all branches of medicine also raise the question, whether everything that is technically possible ought to be executed under all conceivable circumstances, or whether we have to introduce limitations, and if so, according to which criteria.

Furthermore, both medical ethics and the law, at least in the entire western world, have adopted the principle of the patient's right to privacy and self-determination. This significantly changes the traditional approaches to medical decision making, and also considerably, influences the doctor-to-patient relationship, which was the primary object of Cushing's common devotion.

Finally, the increase in internationalisation during the last decades, due to the growing number of international journals and congresses and other modern methodes of communication, means that all new developments and advances, and all knowledge in medicine reach the farthest corners of the world very rapidly. But, this also brings together many different cultures and religions, sometimes with enormously diverse views on fundamental matters like disease, death, euthanasia, abortion, in vitro fertilization, genetic engineering and organ transplantation. As it is unlikely that we will ever reach full agreement between these cultures and religions, it is even more unlikely that we will achieve a common worldwide opinion on medical moral standards. One even can encounter more conflicting opinions on these matters within one particular country or in one particular culture than between the different cultures and different religions.

This growing complexity of medical practice has increased exponentially, together with the technical developments in medicine, during the last few decades. It is highly likely that this complexity will increase even further and at least at the same rate in the next few years. This not only creates a challenge for those who wish to philosophise on medical ethics and moral standards for the future, but also seems to be an occupational hazard in itself. On the other hand, if we continue developing new medical opportunities in future, and no doubt we will, we also bear the responsibility for drawing up the ethical standards, so that we can safely apply the new achievements to the benefit of our patients. The very least we must do, therefore, is to provide ourselves with a moral framework, which will help us to make sound decisions even in difficult or unusual circumstances. One might add this obligation to Cushing's definition of common devotion.

These considerations hold for neurological surgery to an even greater extent than for many other medical specialties. The first reason for this is that neurosurgeons and neurologists are involved, more than other specialists, in the management of large numbers of critically ill patients, many of whom have faulty judgement or impaired consciousness as a consequence of their illnesses. In this respect, Langfitt pointed out: "More than others, neurosurgeons and neurologists are taught to know: – when brain function is so impaired that individuals are no longer able to weigh the choices available to them and are therefore no longer competent to manage their own affairs including decisions about life and death; – when the brain is irreversibly damaged, based on an analysis of the nature and extent of the brain insult and knowledge from personal experience and the scientific literature on the likelihood of survival, and useful survival, if the patient is kept alive; – and finally, when the brain is dead." [2] The second reason, that the neurosurgeon in particular is involved in moral considerations is, that, even if the patient is competent of making his own decisions and of providing informed consent, he will never be able to calculate all the possible consequences of his choice. The neurosurgeon will always keep the full responsibility for his advice and his action, in which the patient has to place his trust. With respect to this responsibility of the neurosurgeon, Paul Bucy stated in an Editorial in Surgical Neurology some twenty years ago: "The responsibility of performing operations which can improve or ruin the intellect, the

ability to speak and understand, to walk, to run and to feel, is one not shared by those in any other field of medicine". [3] These two factors: the severity of the patient's illness, almost always including mental impairment, and the far-reaching consequences of neurosurgical actions, put a special responsibility on the neurosurgeons' shoulders. New developments in neurosurgery may also easily touch the quality of human life. And therefore, neurosurgeons, as no others, have the bounden duty to maintain an overall view of these developments in their own specialty and to draw up the ethical standards for their actions, as mentioned before.

These thoughts have been the leitmotiv for putting together this symposium on "Neurosurgery and Medical Ethics". Of course, we cannot speak of the "Ethics of Neurosurgery". And we must realize that, even in a like-minded intellectual group as the Academia Eurasiana Neurochirurgica, it is absolutely impossible to aim for a consensus on ethical standards in neurological surgery. But we have to see ourselves living in a multicultural society, placed in an always changing doctor-to-doctor and doctor-to-patient relationship. And therefore, we at least have to be informed about different views of medical ethics for a good mutual understanding and respect. During this symposium, we first will hear about the moral backgrounds of medical ethics from the perspective of some of the most important cultures and religions in Asia and Europe. Then, the ethical aspects in different fields of neurosurgical practice will be discussed. And finally, we will have some contributions on teaching in moral attitude and ethical behaviour. We may hope, that this symposium will give us a broader perception of medical ethics in general, and will offer us an ethical framework to fulfil the commitments and expectations in our daily practice.

### References

1. Cushing H (1926, 1928) Consecratio medici. Graduation address, Jefferson Medical College, Philadelphia, Boston, Little, Brown, and Company
2. Langfitt TW (1989) Critical care: when is enough enough? In: PMcL Black (ed) Williams and Wilkins, Baltimore. Clin Neurosurg 35: 15–28
3. Bucy PC (1978) Queen of surgical arts. Editorial. Surg Neurol 10: 317

Correspondence: H. August van Alphen, M.D., Ph.D., Hogerlustlaan 57, 1191 CL Ouderkerk a/d Amstel, The Netherlands.

Acta Neurochir (1999) [Suppl] 74: 17–27
© Springer-Verlag 1999

# Medical Ethics from the Muslim Perspective

A. van Bommel, Imam

Van de Sande Bakhuyzenstraat, Hilversum, The Netherlands

## Introduction

In view of everything written about freedom of religion in the national law of most European countries, international law and declarations of human rights, Muslims are free to take autonomous decisions about bio-ethical problems. However, autonomy as a right does not mean that Muslim individuals have the medical and ethical information at their disposal which could enable them to take the right decisions. *The Universal Islamic Declaration of Human Rights* states in its first article, *Right to Life*: Human life is sacred and inviolable and every effort shall be made to protect it. In particular no one shall be exposed to injury or death, except under the authority of the Law. Just as in life, so also after death, the sanctity of a person's body is handled with due solemnity.

In about 47 countries Islam forms the background of religious and cultural life. In most of these countries we see differences in the strained relationships between state, Muslimscholars and the population. Within this triangle of power the influence of Islamic revelation and prophethood changes and I would like to describe *Shari'ah*, or Islamic Law, as it is sometimes translated, as a collective ethical (sub)consciousness of the Muslim masses. Apart from this we can observe an interaction of influences between western ethical thought and developing Muslim self consciousness in this field.

The tendency of many Muslims to go back to the golden age of Islam, the time of the Prophet, has led many observers to believe that Islam became fossilized as a result of the strict clinging to externals. But to show that fundamentalists are, contrary to the spirit of the Prophet or his immediate followers, eternalizing the decisions given on concrete cases, we have to go back to that time to demasque the fiction of the closing of the door of *ijtihâd*, or Islamic source-interpretation by individual reasoning. We have to draw the attention of our co-religionists and the adherents of other religions to the Qur'anic statement: *"God changes not what is in a people, until they change what is in themselves" (13:12)*.

Another verse of the Qur'an: *"Whatever good befalls you is from God and whatever of evil befalls you is from yourself" (4:79)*, also means that we sometimes can change our conditions with our own hands. As the Qur'an shows us, the image of man is composed of several qualities. Stewardship, soul, natural inclination to worship God and free will are some of the most important. To make clear how this *Qur'anic human being* sees himself, I quote an example from a book on healing, written by a Muslim mystic:

"What is a human being? How did it come into existence? How is it sustained in existence? And what is the purpose of human life? Without understanding the answers to these questions (or at least the questions), we can never have a satisfactory knowledge of the real type of health we should be seeking. For without any criteria for what constitutes the proper functioning of a human being, how can we say that it even matters whether we are ill or well? Just because something feels 'good' does not necessarily mean it is of ultimate benefit to us. And conversely, simply because at the moment we seem to have pain, we cannot dismiss the experience as 'bad', unless we understand how and what the result of these momentary sensations will be. For the Qur'an says: *'There may be a thing decreed for you that you do not like, that is good for you; and things that you like, that are not good for you' (2:216)*. The well known scholar and mystic al-Ghazali expressed this idea as follows: 'Illness is one of the forms of experience by which humans arrive at a knowledge of God;

as He says, 'Illnesses are My servants which I attach to My chosen friends'."[1] A way of giving meaning to illness.

One thing is evident: human being means ethical being in the Qur'an. In this presentation I will try to investigate some of the legal, ethical and methaphysical sources by which a Muslim is influenced and enabled to take ethical decisions.

## Ethics

The main sources to understand the ethics of Islam are the Qur'an (revelation), the Ahadith (traditions), and the interpretative literature derived from them. One of our methods could be that we move from deduction to induction: that is, to draw general principles and conclusions from specific rules and categories. Apart from drawing general ethical principles from the specific rulings of the Qur'an, we also need to analyse contemporary reality using the basic concepts of Islam. Both of these concepts work as operators for analysing modern problems and evolving Islamically inspired solutions to them. Concepts like istislah (public interest) and istihsân (equity) mean to take in hand the keys to disclose among others, the Muslim theories about ecology, economy, politics and technology.

Islamic ethics splits into deontology and utilism and the interaction of these two disciplines is recognizable within the Islamic discipline of akhlaq (morality, ethics) and in harmony with its epistemological theory. The Muslim community in the West is waking up to the fact that it struggles with the answers to the material and spiritual questions of an over-infrastructurised and over-rationalised society. Western medical ethics and technology are a part of the social industry. The issues of health and disease have come under sharp focus as questions of cultural values. The definitions of health and disease may ultimately shape the entire corpus of medical practice. As a community Muslims do not yet have a deeper understanding of the ideas of the contemporary Muslim scholars in the field of medical ethics, nor of the latest findings in the West. Some independent thinkers present Islam as an ethical and social system. To circumscribe Islam with the yardstick of civics may give some limitations, although reading through the Qur'an 'diagonally' we can actually find the contours of a complete ethical system – a

method which also offers a more comprehensive and integrated picture of Islam as a whole. Exaggerating the importance of 'being ethical' sometimes creates the illusion of misplaced moral and spiritual superiority feelings and possibly leads to neglect of the daily social-political reality. In Islam ethics have a purpose. They serve to form social and individual behaviour. But speculating about implementing the orthopraxis sometimes replaces functionality by devotion, power by moral behaviour and courageous creativity by righteousness. Piety, morality, and justice are some of the tools of Islam, but are not goals in themselves. Ethics are our compass but they are not the end of the journey[2].

## Respect for the Dignity of Human Life: Four Ethical Principles

The Islamic Medical Code of Ethics states that therapeusis is a noble profession. God honoured it by making it the miracle of Jesus, son of Mary. Abraham, enumerating his Creator's gifts to him, included: "... and if I fall ill He cures me". This seems to be in harmony with the preamble describing the ethical background of the considerations taking place before the decision-making process of giving or withholding life by prolonging medical treatment.

In caring for patients, doctors and other health care professionals, as individuals and as representatives of their profession, should act with respect for human life and with integrity in providing medical treatment with certain norms of care and concern. Despite widely diverse national, cultural, religious and political traditions, four prima facie moral principles summarise these norms[3].

---

[1] Shaykh Hakim Moinuddin Chisti (1991) The Book of Sufi Healing, Inner Traditions International, Vermont, p 11

[2] Acknowledgements to Ziauddin Sardar
[3] The internationally well known Principles of Biomedical Ethics of Beauchamp/Childress (1989) has, as much as anything else, contributed to the cross cultural discours about medical ethics. One of the goals is to come to a reflective equilibrium from the morals shared by the other members of the world community. 'Of particular importance are questions concerning the cultural assumptions that inform our beliefs about the significance and relevance of bio-ethics for the art and practice of healing. The intercultural bio-ethics discourse is enhanced when there is at least minimal agreement over the process of moral reasoning and a shared understanding about the context of particular medical practices. Finally, respect for cultural differences must be maintained without sacrificing the value placed on basic human rights. From: Intercultural Reasoning: the Challenge for International Bioethics, Patricia Marshall, David C. Thomasma, Jurrit Bergsma (1994) Cambridge Quarterly of Healthcare Ethics 3: 321–328

## Autonomy

The first human being used his free will to disobey his Creator. You cannot be more autonomous, I would say. The integrity of human beings and their freedom of will and acting is expressed by the Qur'an: *"We offered the trust to the heavens and the earth and the mountains, but they refused to carry it and were afraid of it; and man carried it. Surely he is sinful, very foolish" (33:72)*.

That is why God, according to the Qur'an, breathed into him from His spirit and made the angels bow to the first human being (2: 30–31). To believe is a free act of men: *"... so let whosoever will believe, and let whosoever will disbelieve ..." (18:29)*, says the Qur'an. *"Surely We guided him upon the way wether he be thankful or unthankful" (76:3)*. In this verse unbelief is called unthankfulness: life is a blessing for which one is to be thankful. Jalaluddin Rumi said: "Free will is the endeavour to thank God for His beneficence".

The Qur'an puts its trust in the rational power of human beings to distinguish between truth and falsehood: *"No compulsion is there in religion. Rectitude has become clear from error" (2:256)*. Our next question should be: is this Qur'anic autonomous human being authorized and able to dispose when decisions about life and death have to be taken? "Officially it is all very clear", says drs. D. P. Touwen, ethicist of the Dutch Care Federation, in her article in the daily *Trouw*, "if it is about a decision on medical treatment, yes or no, than the practitioner gives all the relevant information to the patient and it is up to the patient to decide what he wants".

Of course one can pose many open questions here. Does the human body participate in human dignity and will this feeling of wholeness dictate the autonomous decision? Is it the reasonableness of the medical treatment itself or is it the agreement of the patient that forms the decisive ground for justification of the eventual violation of the corporal integrity. For Muslims experiencing corporality also has a methaphysical dimension. And although Islam wants to protect the body's integrity, it also wants to sacrifice it for a higher value. Like the well-being of the community in general and saving life in particular[4]. 'Human life is sacred ... and should not be wilfully taken except upon the in-

dications specified in Islamic Jurisprudence, all of which are outside the domain of the Medical Profession'. 'A doctor shall not take away life, even when motivated by mercy...' (Islamic Code of Medical Ethics).

While there is a strong moral reserve, based on respect for human dignity during its lifetime and even after, because of the expectation of the resurrection and responsibility in front of the Creator[5] – that blocks the removal of organs after death, Islamic ethics also recognizes several competing principles that, under certain circumstances, can bracket this reservation. For a Muslim patient absolute autonomy is very rare, there will be a feeling of responsibility towards God, and he or she lives in a social coherence, in which influences of the imam and relatives play their roles. Muslims feel very strongly that it is Allah Who does the actual healing, the doctor being only the agent for the will of Allah. This consciousness is based on the Qur'anic verse: *"If Allah touch you with affliction, none can remove it but He" (6:17)*.

## Non-Maleficence (Avoid Harm)

The infliction or risking of harm to others, including the risks of medical practice, can only be justified by the pursuit of other moral values – principally, in the case of medical practice, benefits to patients sufficient to outweigh the harm. Medical practitioners generally see this principle as linked to the principle of beneficence. Indeed, most would say they are two sides of the same coin. The Islamic point of view: 'No harm shall be inflicted or reciprocated in Islam'[6]. Many Muslim scholars consider the above mentioned concept of *istihsan* to be a method of seeking facility and ease in legal injuctions. This is a cardinal principle in religion which is enunciated in the Qur'an, where we read: *'God desires ease for you, and desires not hardship for you ...'* (2:185).

One prophetic tradition reads: 'The best of your re-

---

[4] '... if anyone saves a life, it shall be as though he had saved the lives of all mankind' (5:32)

[5] 'Is, then, He who has created the heavens and the earth not able to create anew the like of those who have died?' (36:81) And: "Does man think that we cannot resurrect him and bring his bones together again? Yea indeed, we are able to make whole his very fingertips!' 75: 3–4

[6] Based on the musnad Hadith (tradition with a complete chain of authorities from the narrator to the Prophet himself): 'there should be neither harming nor reciprocating harm'. (Ibn Mâjah, Imam Malik, etc)

ligion is that what brings ease to the people'. The Qur'an shows doing good as the opposite of inflicting harm: '... *and whosoever has done an atom's weight of good shall see it, and whosoever has done an atom's weight of evil shall see it' (99:8).*

Philosophically and ethically it may be more important to abstain from doing harm. To withhold a medicine from a patient can never be justified. The Islamic Code of Medical Ethics says: 'Wherever welfare is found, there exists the statute of God'. According to some of the Muslim scholars the principle of non-maleficence meant a justification for decisions to forgo life-prolonging medical treatment, when continuation of treatment would damage the patient. Another example is in the discussion about organ transplantion. Although there is no codification of fatâwâ yet, the majority of Muslim scholars interpreted the general rulings, found in Qur'ân and Ahadith in favour of new medical techniques. For the transplant of organs as for certain other decisions, the two main basic rules are: *Necessity has no law* and *Necessities render the prohibited permitted,* mainly based on the verse of the Qurân: '... *but if one is driven by necessity – neither coveting it nor exceeding his immediate need – no sin shall be upon him: for, behold, God is much-forgiving, a dispenser of grace' (2:173).*

Here the lesser harm, that will be the result of the operation of the organdonor, is accepted because of prevention of a greater harm if we do not transplant the organ into the patient. The same comparison has been made between the particular harm done to the donor, and public harm done to society at large, because the population wants to feel safe and secure, knowing there is a possibility to survive lethal illnesses.

## Beneficence (Do Good)

The encouragement to do good is manifest on many pages of the Qur'an in many different meanings, depending on the context. "... *and whatever good you may do, God has knowledge of it" (2:215).* Truthfulness, unconditioned goodness and mercy for the poor and destitute are among the qualities that belong to the blessed state that result from the performance of unselfish behaviour. "... *those who love all that come to them in search of refuge, and who harbour in their hearts no grudge for whatever the others may have been given, but rather give them preference over themselves, even though poverty be their own lot: for, such as from their*

*own covetousness are saved – it is they, they that shall attain to a happy state!" (59:9).*

By beneficence is meant here acting rightly by offering comfort to the poor, to the less fortunate, and to those of our brethren in the community who have fallen on evil days ... owing to natural handicaps, orphanhood, illness, misfortune, or ignorance, among other causes[7].

Within the different schools of thought different opinions exist, about the concepts of good and evil. For example between the Ash'arite- and the Mu'tazilaschools.

'For, whereas the latter held that man can determine rationally what is good and evil, prior to Revelation, the Ash'arites adhered to a strict voluntarist ethics. Good is what God has prescribed, evil what He has prohibited. In keeping with this voluntarist thesis, they were reluctant to admit that any merit attached to that type of rational knowledge which is attainable through unaided reason. God's power and sovereignty are such that the very meaning of justice and injustice is bound up with His arbitrary decrees. Apart from those decrees, justice and injustice, good and evil, have no meaning whatsoever. Thus God is not compelled, as the Mu'tazila had argued, to take note of moral or religious interests, so to speak, but is entirely free to punish the innocent and remit the sins of the wicked. And had He so desired, He could have created a universe entirely different from the one which He has in fact created, or refrained from creating this universe or any part of it altogether'[8].

According to islamic belief, God is the Healer. But this does not mean that Muslims will sit and wait till they will be healed by prayer or that they refuse medical treatment, because it would be against the will of God. The prophet Ibrahim says in the Qur'an: '*And when I sicken, then He healeth me'* (26:80). The laws of the world that God created are such that each result has its cause. Healing therefore is a result which has a cause. This is why the Prophet said: 'O servants of Allah, seek the cure, because Allah did not create a disease without creating its cure, except for one disease'.

'What is that?' asked his companions. He said:

---

[7] Abdul-Rahman Azzam (1979) The Eternal Message of Muhammad, Quartet Books, London, p 89

[8] Majid Fakhry (1983) A History of Islamic Philosophy, 2nd edn. Columbia University Press, Longman

senility. In another version he said: '... except for the toxic which is death'.

So, to seek the cure: i.e. medical scientific research, is viewed upon as an act of worship and a part of beneficence. As well as, for example, the donation of body parts, is looked upon as being a social duty for the Muslim community, technically called *Fard al-kifâya*: a task that will be taken from the shoulders of the rest of the community if a sufficient nummer of people implement this duty.

## Justice

God is just; all that He does aims at what is best for His creation; He does not desire evil and does not ordain it. He has nothing to do with man's evil deeds; all human actions result from man's free will. Man will be rewarded for his good deeds and punished for his evil ones. From the Qur'anic point of view: *'Surely, God enjoins justice ...' (16 : 90); 'make peace between them with justice' (49 : 9).*

*'... and shaped thy nature in just proportions ...' (82 : 7).* Which means, 'made thee proportionate', i.e. a being subject to physical needs and emotional urges, and at the same time endowed with intellectual and spiritual perceptions: in other words, a being in whom there is no *inherent* conflict between the demands of the spirit and the flesh since both these aspects of the human condition are 'God-willed' and, therefore morally justified.

Like understanding beneficence by comparing it with its opposite we should compare *adl* with *zulm*. *Zulm* is the seminal concept of Islam which has been thoroughly internalised in Islamic history and which even today serves as the pivot of Muslim political and moral conscience. *Zulm* is a negative concept implying the absence of justice and order. The verb *zalama* further implies the act of falsification: to commit any wrongful act and hide, as it were, the face of compassion, equity and justice.

Human beings are entitled to justice:

*"Be ever steadfast in upholding equity, bearing witness to the truth for the sake of God, even though it be against your own selves or your parents and kinsfolk ..." (4 : 135).*

*"... and when you judge between the people, that you judge with justice" (4 : 58).*

*"... and let not hatred of any people seduce you that ye deal not justly. Deal justly that is nearer to your duty" (5 : 8).*

Whatever its moral and ethical connotations, the concept of *zulm an-nafs*, for instance, is eminently reflective and invites man to ponder the troubles and discontent of his existence. Muslim thinkers may and should fruitfully employ the notion of *zulm an-nafs;* 'self-wronging self'[9].

## Fatâwâ

Islam is not a church and has no church-organization with legislative power. The so-called Islamic law or shari'ah is not based on the legal authority of a churchlike organization or institute, nor on any government that recognizes Islam as the religion of state. Maybe we could interpret shari'ah as being the collective ethical subconscious of the ummah.

Since 1981 international conferences on Islamic Medical Ethics frequently take place in several Muslim countries, especially in Kuwait. In the literature resulting from these conferences, an interaction takes place between practitioners, medical scientists and juridical-theologians, to introduce this term for Muslim religious scholars. The process of questioning on these occasions is called *istiftâ* (inquiry), and the answer-formulating process by juridical theologians and ethicists is called *iftâ*, and the product is called *fatwâ* (responsum).

Somebody once asked the prophet: 'What is virtue?' to which he replied 'Virtue is that in which the heart becomes peaceful'. Not so much an external legal opinion, a *fatwâ* is a thing that matters, but: 'Ask your heart for a *fatwâ*'.

Most of the Muslim scholars who produce *fatâwâ* do not interpret directly from the sources but, rather, compare with and build on the texts of their colleages or quote authorities and existing precedents in support of their contention. Seldom do you find an independent *fatwâ*. The well-known Iraqi scholar, Dr. Ala'ed-din Kharofa, Professor of Shari'ah, Kulliyah of Laws, International Islamic University of Malaysia, is very careful in his formulation when dealing with Post Mortem in Islam: 'A fatwa (verdict) of Shaikh Yusuf Nasr al-Dajawi in Egypt says: 'We do not have in jurisprudence books or any satisfactory statement on the topic. Someone might think that it is forbidden by the

---

[9] Ziauddin Sardar (1989) An early Crescent. The Future of Knowledge and the Environment of Islam; Parvez Manzoor S, The Crisis of Muslim thought and the Future of the Ummah, pp 85–86

Islamic law which honours the human being and encourages giving him due respect and forbids abusing them. But he who knows about the spirit of *shari'ah* and how it strives to realise man's interests and its aims, will know that it always draws a balance between benefit and damage and draws its judgement on the basis of stronger evidence in accordance with requirements of wisdom and correct study. So we must have far sighted views which will take into account the stronger benefit which agrees with the spirit of the law which is good for every place and every time and which guarantees well being and happiness in this world as well as in the Hereafter. Thus we feel that post-mortem examination can be seen to be necessary in certain situations ...'[10]

The strength of a legal rule is to a large extent determined by the language in which it is communicated. To distinguish the clear from the ambiguous and to determine the degrees of clarity/ambiguity in words also helps the jurist in his efforts at resolving instances of conflict in the law. When the *mujtahid* is engaged in the deduction of rules from indications which often amount to no more than probabilities, some of his conclusions may turn out to be at odds with others. *Ijtihâd* is therefore not only in need of comprehending the language of the law, but also needs a methodology and guidelines with which to resolve instances of conflict in its conclusions. (Kamali, 1991)

In the decision making process the autonomy of Muslim ethicists seems as critical and desirable as the autonomy of the Muslim patient.

There are only a few independent Muslim scholars who dare to write down their opinions independently from the recognized authorites. Sometimes this meant they had to live in exile.

Not every *fatwâ* is absolute. Sometimes people council with several mufti's in different countries and choose the most convenient, the most convincing, or the most logical, or the most affirmed answer. Sometimes the well-known process of wanting to hear what you already ought to know takes place. For this reason the position of the *mufti* or *mujtahid* is one of very heavy responsibility, with many conditions to fulfil.

Next to mastering all the basic sciences of Islam, he should be of sound mind and proper conduct and capable of comprehending systematically and of dis-

cernment. Knowledge of the rules of interpretations is essential to the proper understanding of a legal text.

Although the bulk of twentieth-century Muslim literature represents imitative conformism in the fields of religion, politics and economics, in the fields of ethics there is constant development. We most probably can even speak of the dynamics of ethics. When we study the Islamic medical ethics, one of the few sources of information is the above mentioned *fatâwâ*-literature. Next to the vast amounts of *responsa* from previous centuries, this literature is formed by a large amount of contemporary legal responses, a mirror of the dialogue between the laymen and the experts of *shari'ah*. In the libraries of the big cities of the Muslim world, such as Cairo, Riyadh, Makka, Fez, etc., we can find these standardised collections of *Fatâwâ*.

In many of the Muslim countries where the Arabic language is not spoken, selections of these *fatâwâ* are available in Indonesian, Turkish or other languages. In English you can find *fatâwâ* in concise selections, manuals and several newspapers and magazines under specific headings, such as Arabic newspapers and magazines. One of the problems of investigating *fatâwâ* literature is the status of the *fatwâ* to which you are referring.

Another problem is that, although most *fatâwâ* are the product of communication – in the question/answer style that has existed already for centuries – it is not communicative itself. Language-wise, *fatâwâ*-literature does not enter into dialogue with, nor does it explain itself to young Muslims who live in the USA or northern Europe, nor the new Muslims or non-Muslims.

Arabic is the liturgical as well as the scientific language and also the *lingua franca* of Islam. For young people who do not master this language and the terminology of Islamic jurisprudence there is a double language problem.

The last one or two decennia some of the 'travelling Muslim scholars' have tried to develop *Fatâwâ*-literature, taking into account the Muslim presence in the West as a minority. Classical sources of jurisprudence are dealing with Muslim majorities and *dhimmî*'s (non-Muslim citizens) in area's predominantly inhabited by Muslims. Nowadays, Muslim scholars should consider this change of position vice versa. Especially since the Muslim youth seems to take a distance from the ethical and methaphysical message of Islam, because of a lack of pedagogical and didactical communication towards them.

---

[10] The Journal of the Federation of Islamic Medical Associations (FIMA), vol 1, no 1, (1996) pp 103–104

## Aesculapian Authority

Ethical values are universal but are deeply embedded in cultural contexts[11]. Each culture has its own conception of health and disease and its own approach to healing, therapy and recovery. In every community medicine, like religion and law, has the power to determine what is normal, proper or desirable. It also has the authority to declare whether somebody is ill or not, or to refuse the social recognition of his pain, invalidity or even death. Morality is as indivisibly connected with disease as it is with crime or sin. The interpretation of ethical values is also determined by the resources that are available to individuals, families and communities. The original limited power of the traditional healer has grown tremendously when we speak of the medical specialist in Western societies. Western medicine always wanted to stay out of the power structure of law and religion, and now rules in many categories of society in which many of the social labels are placed in the realm of medical specialists to such a degree that many aberrations have a medical name. Since the ethical component in medical diagnosis is not very clear anymore medical specialists have received almost totalitarian power. At the other hand Muslims living in northern Europe admire the prevailing system of justice in the western world, which has provided equity and access to health services. Switches from one political and economic system to the other, are a restraining influence on the social progress which most of the Muslim countries are in need of, and we still have to reach a level of development where ethical concerns can assume a central position.

In July 1995, a one/day conference on cross-cultural perspectives in healthcare ethics was organized in the city of Utrecht, by the Care Federation, in which the subject of discussion, "Autonomy of Patients", was introduced by John M. Stanley, who is Edward F. Mielke Professor of Ethics in Medicine, Science and Society at Lawrence University and the director of the Lawrence University Program in Biomedical Ethics. One of the visions brought forward was that knowledge and science are value-free and beyond all cultural differences and differences of opinion: the medical specialist can undisputedly make the right decision for his patient. The patient will always agree with his

practitioner after receiving the right knowledge from him.

Another approach toward the patient's autonomy could be that of a human being with more than only medical importance, as one of the participants of the conference pointed out. She asked what was wrong with alternative healing. It is not the medical technological care for one ill part of the body that is most important in a healing process but the attention for the human being as a whole.

This appears to be close to the idea of Islamic healing in certain aspects. However, the problem with the holistic approach is that of the vanished moral dimension of being. The idea of alternative modes of health care is imported from an environment that forms an affirmation with these alternatives in a dynamic equilibrium, but one should question if it will work in the big cities of Europe and the USA. The mere emergence of these attitudes toward health care could be an indication of a pathology of conventional medicine.

Finally there is the idea in which patient and practitioner stand together for a theological task. Muslim consider God to be the Healer with the medical specialist only an instrument of God during the process of healing. With this belief the patient continues to hope for a miracle and will not accept a doctor's statement: 'I cannot do anything for you anymore.'

The practitioner will do a good job if he stands besides his patient. And the patient will trust him most if he actually feels himself an instrument of God. It was interesting to see and hear that some of the participants regarded this last approach as more or less irrational.

The Islamic Medical Code states:

'The doctor shall do his best that what remains of the life of an incurable patient will be spent under good care, moral support and freedom from pain and misery. Euthanasia, or mercy killing of a terminal patient is not allowed within the borders of shari'ah because that should be ignorance of Gods ability to perform miracles. But also because it interferes with God's conclusive control over life and death. As the situation is now, there are no precedents in Islamic Jurisprudence that say otherwise'.

When you talk to people visiting a member of the family in intensive care you will see them gape in admiration at the supertechnology of that room, whatever their cultural background may be, and this is understandable because the longing for miracles is deep within every patient and every loving member

---

[11] Principles of Health Care Ethics (1994) In: Raanan Gillon (ed) chapter: Islam and the Four Principles: a Pakistani View, Dr. Zaki Hasan, John Wiley

of his family. 'Whoever does not believe in miracles, is not a realist', says a Jewish proverb.

## The Sanctity of Human Life

The Qur'an says, *"... that whoso slays a soul not to retaliate for a soul slain, nor for corruption done in the land, shall be as if he had slain mankind altogether; and whoso gives life to a soul, shall be as if he had given life to mankind altogether" (5:32)*.

'Human life is sacred ... and should not be wilfully taken except upon the indications specified in Islamic Jurisprudence, all of which are outside the domain of the Medical Profession' (Islamic Code of Medical Ethics).

'A doctor shall not take away life, even when motivated by mercy. This is prohibited because this is not one of the legitimate indications for killing'. Direct guidance in this respect is given by the Prophet's tradition: 'In old times there was a man with an ailment, he was in such anguish that it taxed his endurance. He cut his wrist with a knife and bled to death. God was displeased and said: My servant hastened his end himself. . I deny him paradise'.

To enable us to understand the arguments that follow, we should first make a short excursion into the Islamic vision on death. In The Islamic Code of Ethics there is the argument that '... mercy-killing like suicide finds no support except in the atheistic way of thinking which believes that our lives on this earth are followed by void'. This is in contrast with the Qur'anic position which says that death is not the end of life. It is only the appointed time (*adjal*), decreed by God, whereby the period of man's testing in this world is concluded.

The post mortem fate of man finds its cause in the action of the individual and the mercy of God. Eternal happiness or damnation is now the question which each person is required to ask himself and to which no one can reply with certainty.

The Islamic conception of death results from a definition of the soul and of life, one vital and the other thinking: *rûh* and *nafs*. *Nafs* has the sense of self in its most conscious and permanent state. *Rûh* is the principle of life which proceeds from God and is enlivened and given substance by Him[12].

---

[12] Lemma. Mawt, the Encyclopaedia of Islam, new edn. Brill, Leiden

Birth and death are divine degrees. Parents do not give life. Events are not the cause of death. These are only the intermediaries through which the will of God is realized. This definition of life strongly influences the metaphysical and moral conceptions of Muslims. By affirming that life proceeds from God and that the loins of fathers and the wombs of mothers are only 'repositories', like the Qur'an says (6:98), Islam confers a new significance on the life of the individual and a new perspective on his action. The life of the individual becomes sacred. *'And slay not the soul God has forbidden, except by right' (17:33)*.

The process described here by the Qur'an is that of substituting the notion of the community of faith for that of the community of blood. Islam led the believers to liberate themselves from ascendancy of the clan and to take cognisance of their existence as free and responsible persons. Even though the believers are declared brothers, they are individually responsible for their actions before judges in this world as well as before God on the final day of judgment.

## Euthanasia

It is often forgotten that euthanasia, the medical termination of human life, could only become an important issue after the 'last cares' had been placed within the realm of medical specialists. The ethical dilemmas associated with euthanasia are therefore relatively new. The dilemmas grew almost at the same tempo as supportive care and "high tech" for terminal patients expanded. That is why, according to some scholars, most of the judicial and ethical discourse about the legal and ethical aspects of this type of professional intervention in the process of dying has little value, because it does not touch upon the legal and ethical aspects of the realm of the medical specialist, of which this issue forms the result in the first place. One of the questions is at which moment in the history of medical technical development we should begin to be critical and ethical.

The Qur'an enjoins us to consider life as a right of every human being. '... slay not the soul God has forbidden, except by right ...' (6:151). A tradition of the Prophet reads: 'The greatest sins are to associate something with God and to kill human beings'. In all texts about this subject the Qur'an and the tradition uses the word nafs (soul) in general terms without any indication that citizens belonging to one's own nation or the people of a particular race or religion should not be killed. The injunction applies to all human beings. Medical ethics is not the Philosophical space to deal with discussions about gender change, homosexuality, prostitution, male-female dispositions, prosmiscuous behaviour, it puts the practitioner in the chosen position of being all-merciful without discrimination. If a human being is wounded or ill, it is our duty to get him medical help. If he/she is dying of starvation, it is our duty to feed him. If he is drowning, it is our duty to rescue him. Muslims should regard it as their duty to save every human life.

Suicide or termination of life, or the numerous means through which mercy-killing can be executed, are not mentioned in detail in the *fatâwâ*. In general, it is stated that euthanasia is not allowed because it is considered murder.

Quoting Ibn Hazm, Mrs. Rispler Chaim says in her study of *Islamic Medical Ethics in the Twentieth Century* 'it is interesting that Islamic law does recognize one's desire to die because of an unbearable religious situation or in order to defend one's religion. Bankruptcy and physical pain, however, do not justify one's wish to die'. She also quotes Jalaluddin Umri's *Suicide or Termination of Life*, in which he says; 'Anyone who commits suicide ignores his/her obligation toward his/her relatives. On the other hand, when suicide is meant to release a patient from a malignant and incurable disease, the patient may claim he/she wished to free relatives of the burden of tending a bedridden person'.

Another remarkable statement is found in the Islamic code of Medical Ethics:

'In his defence of life, however, the doctor is well advised to realize his limit and not transgress it. If it is scientifically certain that life cannot be restored, then it is futile to diligently keep on the vegetative state of the patient by heroic means of animation or preserve him by deepfreezing or other artificial methods. It is the process of life that the doctor aims to maintain and not the process of dying. In any case, the doctor shall not take a positive measure to terminate the patient's life'.

Dr. Muhammad Abduljawwad Muhammad argued as follows during the occasion of the Symposium on the Islamic Vision of some Medical Practices, held on April 18, 1987, in Kuwait:

'With respect to euthanasia, the legal ruling in Shari'ah, which kept unchanged until the invention of resuscitive methods and intensive care, stands that is was on no account permissible. It was made equal to intentional homicide. Yet, after the introduction of such methods which were conducive to life prolonga-

tion of fatally diseased patients, determination of the moment of death became imperative. This began in America in 1950 due to disputes among inheritors. Then the succes of Dr. Christian Bernard in 1976 in removing a heart and transplanting it in another patient came to add a new problem which necessitated determination of the moment of death; for the success of this kind of operation requires removal of the heart after brain death and prior to stoppage of circulatory functions. He continues with saying that there is gradation from clinical death to brain death then to biological death and on to cellular death ... which of the death criteria should we adopt ... to the medical aspect it determines when it is permissible to remove some of the organs for transplantation into another body.

Objectivity of research and scientific honesty require me to state, quoting American legal references, that in 1957 Pope Pius XII made permissible removal of the respirator from patients who are in irreversible coma.

This is the same thing concluded by some of our Shari'ah jurists at the present time'.

Dr. Salah al-Ateeqi gathered some cases, which he treated in his paper entitled 'When there is a conflict between Sharia and law: what attitude shall a doctor take?' According to me it is possible to review these cases by analogy with the type of contemplation primary to euthanasia. Males taking decisions about the lives of their wifes and children as well as doctors taking their decisions, had their ethical considerations, with life-and-death questions which have remarkable similarities with the reflections about euthanasia.

1. Some men refuse a male doctor to undertake examination of their women who are in a degree of consanguinity precluding marriage or perform surgical operations on them which may be urgent and cannot be delayed. Does the doctor have the right to carry out the operation in spite of the husband's objection if the female patient is in danger and no female doctor is available? Both from the standpoints of Shari'ah and law the answer is 'yes'. Moreover it is not only the doctors right but also his duty which if not done, the doctor will be held legally delinquent in law and Shari'ah-wise sinful. Does the husband have the right to kill his wife in this way by failing to accept medical assistance from a doctor? The answer to this question is included in the first question and answer; the husband has no right, neither in the law nor in Shari'ah.

2. A child suffers from hydrocephalus. Father refuses

that operation is done within the first days of birth and prefers to let him die rather than to have a son who may have some sort of deformity. The question is: does the father have the right to kill his son in this way, and what is the attitude of Shari'ah and law? Answer: Either in law or Shari'ah, consent of the father is of no consequence and the doctor must perform the operation.

3. During a normal delivery the foetal condition has deteriorated and consequently a Caesarean Section is necessary to save the foetus from death. Yet the father refuses to have the operation performed on his wife, thus sacrificing the child which had an almost certain chance to live if the operation had been undertaken. Does the father have any right to dispose of his son's life with such cruelty, and what is the legal and Shariah attitude? The answer is that the father has no right to act in this way and the attitudes of both law and Shari'ah is that the father's will is of no consequence in such a case and the operation has to be performed'. The Islamic Code of Medical Ethics states in 'The Oath of the Doctor: I swear by God... To be, all the way, an instrument of God's mercy, extending my medical care to near and far, virtuous and sinner, friend and enemy ...'
That is why the decisions of the participants in the Symposium on the Islamic Vision of some Medical Practices, are based on mercy, and the decisions of patients and relatives in the three above mentioned cases are based on ignorance. The main task seems to be to bridge the wide knowledge-gap, between what Islam has to say about it and between healers and patient. This information vacuum could be the main reason why sometimes decisions are made without considering the autonomy of the patient.

Because of the fact that compassion is one of the central themes of Islam and considering some of the openings for discussion mentioned above, we have to ponder the question: is it merciful to prolong life if, also according to the Islamic definition of quality of life, forgoing life-prolonging treatment would be more appropriate, or does not such a situation occur?

## Conclusion

The significance of cultural assumptions regarding the semantics of ethical dialects and the application of biomedical technology make clear that in order to have an inter-cultural and inter-religious understand-

ing we should try to come to a common vocabulary. It is necessary that we – during our struggle for dialogue and global mutual understanding – continue to believe in the crossfertilization of our cultures.

Apart from the momentum of revelation of the Qur'ân and the emergence of the Muslim community, 14 centuries ago, two periods in the history of Islam showed this capacity for cultural blooming, based on intercultural relationships. These were the periods of cooperation between Jews, Christians and Muslims in Bagdad and in Al-Andalus. The debate on medical ethics seems to be dominated by liberal terminology. The liberal moral culture gives importance to the right of selfdetermination, autonomy, the religious culture probably cares more for sanctity and protection of life. Are these two ethical principles of the same importance to us? Sometimes Muslims experience indifference when the secular majority seems to be prepared to put aside all kinds of ethical deliberations based on religion to come quickly to a consensus. The urgency to bring up for discussion the apparent evidences of the established medical and bio-ethical discourse increases when an established moral order is confronted with other cultures and religions, i.e. with other possibilities to experience the human body. (Zwart, 1998)

Consensus on issues may not always be feasible. According to Marshall, Thomasma and Bergsma, minimal agreement must be reached regarding the language, meaning, and value of ethical concepts and processes of moral reasoning. This agreement will require explicit self-critical attention to the meaning of concepts and their cultural context in ways that have not yet been present in the international dialogue. Secondly there should be a commitment to discerning cultural context. Bioethics can be the beneficiaries of the richness that characterises cultural diversity if opportunities are created to experience the challenge of transcultural dialogue. Yet, this challenge will require a new and perhaps uneasy acceptance (for some) of pluralism. Thirdly more serious philosophical work should be done on transcultural structures in human behaviour and existence. One such structure may be that of human rights.

The motivation or aversion, for or against dialogue sometimes is coloured by historical consciousness and the unbalanced economical and political relations between the Muslim world and the West, or more generally by the North-South relationships. The tensions between ideas about individuality and collectivity; personal freedom and joint social responsibility can make up the greater part of the elementary differences. As a Muslim community we have to make a passing manoeuvre, for we have an, at least, twofold responsibility: to communicate towards our own women and children and to participate in the global ethical dialogue.

## References

1. Abdullahi A An-Na'îm, Jerald D Gort, Henry Jansen & HM Vroom (1995) Human Rights and Religious Values, an Uneasy Relationship?, Currents of Encounter, Rodopi BV, Amsterdam
2. Abdullahi Ahmed An-Na'im (1990) Toward an Islamic Reformation, Civil libirties, Human Rights, and International Law, Syracuse University Press, Syracuse, New York
3. Abul Hasan Ali Nadwi (1976) Saviours of Islamic Spirit, Academy of Islamic Research and Publications, P.O. Box 119, Lucknow – 7, India
4. Abdul Haq Ansari (1986) Sufism and Shari'ah, Study of the Religious Thought of an Oustanding Sufi and a Great Renovator of Islam, Shaykh Ahmad Sirhindî (1564–1624), Islamic Foundation, Leicester
5. Avicenna (1991) Leerdicht der Geneeskunst, Uitg Boom, Meppel/Amsterdam (Didactic Poem on Medicine)
6. Mohammed Ali Albar, Islamic View on Organ Transplantation, King Fahd Medical Research Centre, King Abdulaziz University, Jeddah, P.O. Box 2631, Jeddah, 21641
7. Approaches to Health Care Ethics (1994) Ranaan Gillon (ed) John Wiley & Sons Ltd
8. A. van Bommel (1993) Islam en Ethiek in de Gezondheidszorg
9. Rispler-Chaim V (1993) Islamic Medical Ethics in the Twentieth Century
10. Majid Fakhry (1983) A History of Islamic Philosophy, 2nd edn. Columbia University Press, Longman
11. Majid Fakhry (1991) Ethical Theories in Islam, EJ Brill
12. Hassan Hathout (1984) Topics in Islamic Medicine (1st edn) International Organisation of Islamic Medicine, Kuwait
13. Maragaretha T Heemskerk (1995) Pain and Compensation in Mu'tazilite Doctrine, Abd al-Gabbars Teaching and its Adoption by Mankdîm and by Mattawayh, Nijmegen
14. Mohammad Hashim Kamali (1991) Principles of Islamic Jurisprudence, Islamic Texts Society, Cambridge
15. Pranger D (1997) Islam en Gezondheidszorg, Ambo bv, Baarn
16. Qadir CA, Philosophy and Science in the Islamic World, Routledge, London, New York
17. Fazlur-Rahman (1967) Health and Medicine in the Islamic Tradition, Change and Identity, Crossroad New York
18. Ibn Rushd (1986) Ibn Rushd's Metaphysics, a Translation with Introduction of Ibn Rushd's Commentary on Aristotle's Metaphysics, Book Lâm, Ch. Genequand (ed), EJ Brill
19. Hendrik M Vroom, Jerald D Gort (1997) Holy Scriptures in Judaism, Christianity and Islam, Hermeneutics, Values and Society, Currents of Encounter, Rodopi BV, Amsterdam, Atlanta, GA
20. Mehdi Ha'iri Yazdi, The Principles of Epistemology in Islamic Philosophy, Knowledge by Presence, State University of New York Press
21. Islam (1980) Philosophy and Science, Four Public Lectures Organized by Unesco, The Unesco Press
22. Islamic Code of Medical Ehtics (1981) First International Conference on Islamic Medicine, Kuwait Document
23. The Islamic Vision on some Medical Practices (1987) Full Text of the Symposium on the Islamic Vision of some Medical Practices
24. Bulletin of Islamic Medicine, vol. 5 (1988) Proceeding of the Fifth International Conference on Islamic Medicine, Kuwait
25. Magazine Articles (1986) Munawar Ahmed Anees, the Placebo Effect; Medicine and Metaphysics: the Struggle for Healthy Life-Styles, Ziauddin Sardar; a Life Devoted to Islamic Medicine, Health Science in Early Islam (2 Vols), collected papers by Sami K. Hamarneh, In: Munawar A Anees (ed) Noor Health Foundation and Zahra Publications, 1983/84 (bookreview), Inquiry, Magazine of Events and Ideas, London

Correspondence: Abdulwahid Van Bommel, Imam, Van de Sande Bakhuyzenstraat 68, 1223 CZ Hilversum, The Netherlands.

Acta Neurochir (1999) [Suppl] 74: 29–34
© Springer-Verlag 1999

# Islam and Medical Ethics

**I. Ali Raja**[1] and **M. R. Chaudhry**[2]

[1] Department of Neurosurgery, King Edward Medical College, Lahore, Pakistan
[2] Department of Medicine, Gulberg Hospital Lahore, Pakistan

Medical science continues to make unparalleled advances in technology and skill, the balance between materialism and morality continues to shift towards the attainment of material gains. The other aspect, which continues to be neglected is *ethics*. Ethics simply, is the expression of human values. It speaks of human character and conduct, of the distinction between right and wrong and of one's moral duty and obligations to the community as a whole. Medical ethics thus, pertains to the application of this philosophy in the field of medicine.

Before I talk about medical ethics in the light of Islamic teachings, I feel it necessary to give you a brief introduction about Islam.

God Almighty created the universe including our planet earth. Our planet is inhabited by several creatures including Mankind. The Creator of the Universe created man in His own image. From the very first day the Almighty guided man with His Divine messages in the form of Divine Books and Scrolls for his guidance. After having fully equipped man with all the qualities that the Creator himself desired, he nominated him as "*the most eminent of created things*". As a part of this distinction He blessed him with the power of expression of his mind by speaking, and taught him the art of conversation [1]. This art was bestowed on him so that he could signify the distinction between Good and Evil and Virtue and Vice. Speech is the quality, which distinguishes man from the animals and other creatures.

Likewise another distinctive quality of vital importance bestowed on man is an instrument to judge his dealings and behaviour with his fellows creatures, and his Creator. This is named as "Moral Sense" [2]. By virtue of moral sense he can instinctively distinguish between Good and Evil, truth and falsehood, justice and injustice, right and wrong and this moral sense does not leave him even when he degrades himself to the lowest level of ignorance and negligence.

The inevitable demand of these two distinctive qualities (speech and Moral Sense) is that the method of instruction for man's conscious and voluntary life should be different from other creatures. It does not appear strange that man looks up to his Creator for educating him for fulfilling his responsibility in the Universe. Thus, the Creator made arrangements of Messengers and the Divine Books for education and instruction of man. All the Prophets and the Divine Books brought the same message for mankind, that man should accept God Almighty as his Creator and live his life according to the instructions passed on to him by the Prophets. Muhammad (Peace be upon him) being the last Prophet and Quran being the final and definitive version.

*Prophet Muhammad (PBUH) in his last address delivered the final message of Almighty God. "I have perfected your religion for you and completed my blessing on you and approved Islam as the way of life for you; therefore observe the limits prescribed by the law" [3]*

Now in the light of the teaching of Islam I will discuss the following subjects, which relate to human society.

1. Euthanasia
2. Death
3. Organ Transplantation
4. Homosexuality
5. Aids (HIV Infection)
6. In-vitro Fertilization
7. Cloning

## Euthanasia "Mercy Killing"

*Fourteen hundred years ago, it was revealed in the Holy Quran in Sura Al-Mulk verses 1 and 2 volume 29, and I quote," Full of blessing is He' in Whose hand is the Kingdom of the Universe, and He has power over every thing, Who created death and life that He may try you to see which of you is best in deeds, and He is al-Mighty as well as All Forgiving [4].*

According to this, both life and death are in the hand of Almighty God. The termination of human life is by Allah. He alone determines when a person should die. He also determines the cause of his or her death. When people interfere with that process which Allah has determined, they actually kill. It is interesting to note that euthanasia is defined as *"mercy killing" [5]. This definition acknowledges that it is a killing, and all killing is forbidden in Islam, except as a punishment for certain well defined crimes.* A person who has not committed any of these crimes should not be killed under any circumstances. The reason is that whoever puts him to death actually puts himself in the position of Allah, determining when that person should die. This is an assault on Allah's Authority and is forbidden in Islam.

It is argued that modern medical technology can prolong a patient's life artificially. This questions the definition of life and how it can be prolonged? If it means that people are put on life supporting machines, they will die once the machine is switched off, then that is a very special case. What we have to ask here is whether the brain of such a person who needs a life support machine has ceased to function. If it has, then the life of that person has ended, even though his heart may continue to beat with the help of the machine. Here we are not speaking about euthanasia, but about the definition of life and whether it exists in such a person. There is no doubt that doctors should use every available means to preserve the life of a patient. The use of such life supporting machines is highly beneficial, if it gives the doctors time to administer appropriate treatment. Once it is clear that the patient's brain has ceased to function, then there is no way to bring him back to life. There is no justification for continuing on life supporting machines. The patients' heart will continue to beat without any hope of recovery. The patient has actually died except in name. The switching off of the machine does not in this case fall under "EUTHANASIA".

*The notions of the "right to die with dignity" and "sparing the patient unbearable pain" are not accept-able.* There is no lack of dignity in a person being ill and needing treatment. If he can not control his own body function, then he should be helped with these, to terminate his life is inhuman. To speak of euthanasia in this case is actually suggesting that people are unwilling to help those who are in need of medical and human care. There is no mercy in such a killing. *Even if he makes it clear that he wished to die, and even if his wish is the result of suffering a long, incurable illness, terminating his life is forbidden.*

If people want to be merciful, then they should take good care of such patients. On the other hand, most types of pain can be relieved with appropriate treatment. With the modern advances in medical care, the type of pain which used to be unbearable can easily be reduced or relieved. In a case where it cannot be helped, the patient should be reminded of the fact that he will be rewarded for his pain [6]. If he bears it with resignation and accepts that Allah has determined for him, then his reward will be the forgiveness of his sins. A believer will always be willing to accept such pain for the prize of earning forgiveness and his place in paradise in the world thereafter.

## Death

Death is an abstract noun which may be meaningful to laymen, lawyers, philosophers, and priests but which is very inadequate as a biological description [17]. Death has generally been defined as the cessation of life, or ceasing to exist. Historically, medicine had defined death as an irreversible stoppage of the circulation and respiration. In the early decades of this century and before the present criteria of death, the absent heart beat and respiration were considered synonymous with death. Today, there is an important minority of cases for which we are without an acceptable legal or medical definition of death [18]. The law has always accepted medical definition of death. Thus there is no distinction between the definitions of medical and legal death and the ultimate decision must lie with the doctor, in attendance.

It must be recognised that there is no one moment of death. Man dies in bits and pieces. At the end of life, there is a progression from clinical death – to brain death – to cellular death. The brain death is defined as irreversible cessation of all function of the brain including the brain stem. The determination of brain death is most important at present because of increasing demand for viable organs for transplantation.

Molecular Death follows Biological death after some safe lag period. This interval provides an opportunity for leaving the organs to be transplanted, in the dead body, because they do not undergo disintegration in this period. However, the heart and the kidneys should be removed immediately after Biological death for successful transplantation .

The controversy regarding the definition of death is still continuing; the purpose of death is yet not clear. Life means different things to different human beings [19]. *In Holy Quran a beautiful statement about human life is in Surah AD-DAHR Verses 1 to 4 Volume 29, and I quote, "Has there been a period on man, in endless time, when he was not yet a thing worthy of mention? Indeed, We created man from a mixed sperm drops, to try him, and therefore we made him capable of hearing and seeing. We showed him the ways, whether to be grateful or disbelieving. For the non believer's we have chains and collars and raging fire."*

*And regarding death the Almighty has said [20] in Holy Quran fourteen hundred years ago in Surah AL-A'NAM Verses 93 and 94 Volume 7 and I quote,*

*"Would, that you could see these wicked people, when they are in the agonies of death and the angels would be out-stretching their hands and saying, "Come, yield up your soul; today you shall be awarded a disgraceful torment for the false things you attributed to Allah and for the rebellion you showed against His Revelation." (And Allah will add,) so, you have come before Us all alone, as We created you at first. Now, you have left behind all that we gave to you in the world; and now We do not see with you those intercessors who, you believed, had a share in molding your destinies; all the relations between you have been cut off, and all those, in whom you trusted, have left you in the lurch,".*

Regarding the time of death [21], it is stated in Holy Quran in Surah Al-Qiyamah Verses 26 to 30, Volume 29 and I quote, " When the soul reaches the throat" when the attendants of the patient are disappointed with every remedy and cure, they will say: Let us call at least any chanter who may save him, " the man knows that it is the time of his departure from the world, and the shank is joined to the shank, that will be the day, of driving toward your Lord. In medical terminology its seems to be similar to the definition of biological death.

## Organ Transplantation

Amongst Muslim scholars, organ transplantation has been a subject of controversy for the past 50 years.

The human body consists of the body and its soul. It is created by Almighty God and soul (Ruh) is inspired in it. The human body is lent to man to use it during his life. Though the man is given temporary custody of its body the final possession of the body or any part of it remains in the hand of the Almighty God. After the soul (Ruh) departs from the body by the order of the Almighty, the human body is lifeless and not able to take care of itself. This is the time when the most precious trust of the Universe is returned to its Creator.

*In Surah AT-TIN Verses 1 to 4, Volume 30, God says, "We have created man in the finest of moulds"; meaning that man has been blessed with the best body, and noblest faculties of thought, knowledge and intellect that no other creatures has been blessed with [14].*

*In another place in Holy Quran Surah Bani Isra'il, Verse 70, Volume 15, God Almighty says and I quote " We have honored the sons of Adam and blessed them with conveyance on land and sea and provided them with good and pure things and exalted them above many of our other creatures [15]."*

Islam stresses the honour and the dignity of man- be he alive or dead. A man should be accorded the same respect after his death as he was entitled to when he was alive [16]. *The Holy Prophet Muhammad (PBUH) said, "breaking the bone of a dead person is like breaking the bone of a living person". The Holy Prophet even prohibited siting on the tomb of a dead person.* In Islam the respectful behaviour towards the dead is confined to Muslim as well as non Muslim. The religious leaders and scholars have arrived at a comprehensive and well thought out decision on this matter based on the source of Shari'ah which means the consensus of opinion of religious scholars in the light of Quran, and Hadith (sayings of Holy Prophet), in the intrinsic value of the matters of public interest and the well being of mankind.

Organ transplantation and blood transfusion are in the public interest, of benefit to mankind and not specifically banned in the Islamic teachings. Thus they have been allowed in case the survival of human life is at stake. This is done for the service of community, and serving the needs of the community is not the same as humiliating the enemy. *Blood donation as well as donation of organs is acceptable and is allowed provided it is done for good medical reasons. At the time of donation of organs the donor's security and health should not be put at risk at all.* Transplantation of a organ in a hopeless man with poor prognosis must never be traded for the organ of a healthy man whose own life may be put at risk in an endeavour to save a hopeless man and for the sake of experimentation.

*In a situation, when human donors are not available the consensus of opinion of religious scholars has allowed, transplantation of animal organs. The commercial side of organ donation should be discouraged.*

## Homosexuality

In Holy Quran in Surah Al-Aaraf, Verse 79, 80, 81, 82, 83 and 84 Volume 8 I quote,

*"And We sent Lot as Messenger: Remember that he said to his people, O my people I conveyed the Message of my Lord to you and I did my very best for your good, but I am helpless because you do not like your well wishers and he also said to his people,"* have you become so shameless that you commit such indecent acts as no one committed before you in the world? You gratify your lust with men instead of women: indeed you are people who are transgressors of all limits! But the only answer of his people was no other than to say, " Turn out these people of your habitations for they pose to be very pious." At last we delivered Lot and the members of his household except his wife, who was of those who stayed behind and We rained a rain upon his people, then behold what happened in the end to the guilty ones(7)!*

Reference to the same is also made in Surah Ash Shu'araa, Verses from 160 to 173 Volume 19 [8] and in Surah An-Naml verses from 54 to 58 Volume 19 [9].

After having passed on the divine instructions and the Quranic information to you, I can only say that if adultery is a grave sin, then homosexuality is even worse. All types of human behaviour should be well suited to human nature and human society [10]. Those who indulge in homosexuality do not consider the immoral implications of what they are doing. Homosexuality is an act of humiliation upon the person who is jumped upon. This person loses all dignity and respect. It is against human decency and manners. It has to be treated early. If a person has been spotted, he needs to be treated in a rational way to make him more suitable to fulfil, appreciate and enjoy the qualities which Allah has given him. *I think that the press and Society is responding toward this condemned act in a very strange way, because they participate and promote the so called legal marriages of both homosexual and lesbians.*

## Aids (HIV Infection)

AIDS (Acquired Immuno-deficiency Syndrome) was first recognized in the United States of America in 1981. At present there are approximately one Million HIV infected Americans in the United States.

*Since the recognition of AIDS, the clinical picture, the character of the virus, the social and cultural aspects, the treatment, prognosis and horror have changed all together. One thing that has not changed are the moral aspects of this disease.*

I do not need to go into the detail of the clinical aspects of AIDS, instead I will discuss only the moral aspect of this disease and recommend the ways to rectify the weakness in moral value in the light of the teaching of Islam.

*Fourteen hundred years ago the Holy Prophet of Almighty God had this to say about this disease: "If fahishah or fornication and all kinds of sinful sexual inter-course become rampant and openly practiced without inhibition in any group or nation, Allah will punish them with new epidemics ( Ta'un" and new disease which were not known to their forefathers and earlier generation(11)"*

*Five years ago R. ROOT-BERNSTEIN, of the Free Press, New York said, "If we now go back and ask why AIDS emerged as a problem for gay men only in the past decade or so, despite the acknowledged antiquity of homosexuality itself, the answer becomes clear: AIDS became a problem for homosexual men only when rampant promiscuity, frequent anal forms of intercourse, new and sometimes physically traumatic forms of sex, and the frequent concomitants of drug use, multiple concurrent infections paved the way [12]."*

The Holy Prophet referred to the illegitimate act of homosexuality in which the followers of Prophet Lot were involved and for which that nation was totally destroyed 5000 years ago. *All the scientific evidence indicates that the illegitimate act of homosexuality, fornication and promiscuity are the basic factors in the sustainability and spread of AIDS.*

*Instead of propagating the real knowledge about the prevention of this disease with the missionary spirit and educating the youngsters especially the gay community and proving to them that this type of act indicates their immorality and character bankruptcy, we are boosting their immorality by legalising homosexuality in several countries. The global press and society in general are playing an equally bad role.*

The teaching of morality and the hazards of unnatural acts of homosexuality [13] should be started very early in schools and parents should also take an interest in guarding their children from such vices. Doctors must encourage homosexuals towards a happy matrimony, should give these patients psychotherapy and make them repent of their sins. Instead of encouraging the use of condoms the doctor should condone the promiscuity and fornication, doctors should also involve friends and parents in helping such victims to be drug-free and help them be on the track of legitimate heterosexuality so that they enjoy the pleasure of the opposite sex.

## In VITRO Fertilization

*O ye assembly of Jinn & Men. If it be you can pass beyond, the zones of heavens and the earth, pass ye. Not without authority shall ye be able to pass.*

*Surah Al Rehman (Verse 33, Volume 27) [22]*

*There is no restriction on research and exploration. As a matter of fact it is encouraged as long as it is within the prescribed rules of Allah.*

*The general consensus is that as long as fertilization remains within limits of morality and does not create any social problem it would be permissible i.e. fertilization of wife's Ovum by the husband's sperms.*

## Cloning

The question to which an answer is not clear, Quran prescribes "Ijtehad" which means discussion amongst religious scholars in the light of Quran and Shariah to arrive at a proper conclusion, (Surah Shoora Verse 38 Volume 25) [23]

*In Surah "Rum" Verse 30 Volume 21 [24]. Read as*
*"Do not change creation of Allah,"*
*"Allah's law do not change*
*Final answer to the question of cloning is still awaited from religious scholars.*

## Conclusion

Ladies and gentlemen I took a lot of your precious time to explain the Islamic code of medical ethics which has been described in the last of Allah's Divine revelations. The remedies prescribed in this book for various medical problems we are facing these days are either directly given by Quran or the Hadith. It is food for thought and calls for an in-depth study of the vari-

ous directions given in The Holy Quran. If this is not done, I am afraid we should be prepared to face the consequences of our neglect and disregard of these commandments.

## References

1. God Almighty Imparted the Teaching of Divine Books Including Quran to Man and Gave him the Power of Speech. Holy Quran, Surah Al-Rahman, verse 4, vol 27
2. Almighty God Blessed Man with Reapproaching Self (Conscience) which Stops him from Commiting Evil and makes him Feel Repentant at Doing Wrong, Thinking Wrong and Willing Wrong. Holy Quran, Surah Al- Qiyamah verse 2, vol 29
3. The Last Address of the Holy Prophet Muhammad (PBUH). Holy Quran, Surah Al-Ma'idah, verse 3, vol 6
4. Life and Death has been Created by Almighty God. Holy Quran, Surah Al-Mulk, verses 1–2, vol 29
5. Is Use of Euthanasia Permisible? By Adil Salahi, Islam in perspective section, Arab News P.O.Box 10452 Jeddah 21433 Saudi Arabia
6. Pain and Distress. Holy Quran, Surah Al-Baqarah, verses 155–157, vol 2
7. Homosexuality, Shameless Act of Followers of Prophet Lot (PBUH). Holy Quran, Surah Al-Aaraf, verses 79 to 84, vol 8
8. Homosexuality, Transgressing all Limits of Evil and Sins. Holy Quran, Surah Ash-Shu'araa, verses from 160 to 173, vol 19
9. "Do you Commit Indecency while you see it? Do you Leave Women and Seek Men for the Gratification of your Sexual Desire? The Fact is that you are a People Steeped in Ignorance", Said Prophet Lot. Holy Quran, Surah An-Namal, verses 54 to 58, vol 19
10. Homosexuality. Question and Answers about Islam by Dr. Syed Mutawalli ad-Darsh, Ta-Ha Publishers Ltd. I Wynne Road, London SW9OBB United Kingdom
11. Hadith of the Prophet Muhammad (PBUH). Written in the Forword, of a book, The Aids Crisis: an Islamic Socio-cultural Perspective, Published by The International Institute of Islamic Thought and Civilization (ISTAC) Kaulalumpur, Malaysia, (already given in the text)
12. Statement by Root-Bernstein, in Rethinking Aids (New York the Free Press 1993, P 291) (already given in the text)
13. The Changing Role of Medical and other Anti-Aids Specialists and Moralists. Book-the aids Crisis: an Islamic Socio-cultural perspective. Published by the International Institute of Islamic Thought and Civilization (ISTAC), Kaulalumpur, Malaysia, pp 247–264
14. Man is Created in the Finest of Moulds, Holy Quran, Surah At-Tin, verse 1–4, vol 30
15. Man is Honoured and Exalted Above other Crfatures, Holy Quran, Surah Bani Isra'il, verse 70, vol 15
16. Organ Transplantation. Questions & Answers about Islam. By Syed Mutawalli ad-Darsh, Ta-Ha Publishers Ltd. 1 Wynne Road London SW9 0BB United Kingdom
17. Definition of Death. Current Medical Diagnosis and Treatment (1997) 36 edn, pp 347, 386, 930, 1003
18. Death, its Definition & its Medico-Legal Aspects. Seminar on above subject in Army Medical College Rawalpindi
19. Human Life. Holy Quran, Surah Ad-Dahr, verses 1–4, vol 29
20. Human Death. Holy Quran, Surah Al-A'Nam, verses 93–94, vol 7
21. Time of Death. Holy Quran, Surah Al-Qiyamah, verses 26–30, vol 29

22. O ye assembly of Jinn and man Holy Quran Surah "Rehman", verse 33, vol 27
23. Ijtehad – Holy Quran Surah "Shoora", 42 verse 38, vol 25
24. Do not change the creation of Allah, Holy Quran Surah "Rum", 30 verse 30, vol 21

Correspondence: Iftikhar Ali Raja M.D., Department of Neurosurgery, King Edward Medical College, Gulberg Hospital, Department of Neurosurgery, King Edward Medical College, 4 Gulberg Hospital Complex, 2-Jail Road, Lahore 540194, Pakistan.

Acta Neurochir (1999) [Suppl] 74: 35–46

# Medical Ethics in India: Then and Now

S. K. Pandya

Department of Neurosurgery, Jaslok Hospital & Research Centre, Mumbai, India

## A Brief History of Ancient Indian Medicine

Indian tradition has always sheltered a multiplicity of beliefs and practices. It also reflects the astonishing variation in geography, language and culture across the Indian subcontinent.

Medicine was described in ancient Indian texts as the 'boundless, shoreless, eternal and auspicious science'. Around 1500 BC, Aryan invaders, originating in Central Asia, settled in the northern Indian plains. The Aryans brought with them, in Sanskrit, the beginnings of the *Vedas*. (Whilst Indian historians believe the *vedas* were formulated around 8000 BC, Western historians date them around 1500 BC). The three principal *vedas* were *Rg*, *Sam* and *Yajur*. A later addition was the *Atharva Veda*, the book of the *atharvans* – priests skilled in the performance of rites. It is the principal source for medicine during the early *vedic* period.

The early *Vedic* healers were members of the priestly community. Over the centuries, as religion became increasingly orthodox and rigid, relying on ritual instead of philosophy, priests looked down upon such 'unclean' practices as dissection of dead bodies and surgery. The practice of medicine was then left to individuals outside this elite clan. This was to the advantage of the evolution of medical science in India. The new community of physicians and surgeons, freed from the bonds of orthodoxy, were not averse to learning from whomsoever they could and, in the process, developed a system of medical practice based on observation and experimentation.

With the advent of the schools of Caraka, Susruta and Bhela (800–700 BC), a momentous step was taken from magic and religion to rational therapeutics. A sophisticated, scholastic system evolved, which recorded its findings and teachings in specialised medical textbooks termed *Samhitas* which incorporated empiricism and explanations of observable phenomena. These formed the basis of the ancient Indian science of medicine – *Ayurveda*.

## Ancient Indian Philosophy – The Basis for Ethics

Man and the natural world are seen as manifestations of the eternal *Brahman* (all-pervading consciousness or God). They are constituted of six elements:

– *Atman* – spirit or soul that constitutes the essential self in the person and *Brahman* in the universe;
– Five *mahabhutas* (gross elements: earth, water, fire, air, ether).

*Atman* and the *mahabhutas* are not alien or opposite but parts of an integral whole.

There are three fundamental beliefs in ancient Indian philosophy:

– Each person is being continually reborn – life after life after life (*samsara*).
– What a person does or thinks in each life (*karma*) determines what will be experienced in future lives.
– One's experiences in this life are the result of one's thoughts and actions in past lives.

Increasing the number of good *karmas* and reducing the number of bad *karmas* will automatically cause the person to be reborn higher up in the scale, until he eventually merges with *Brahman* – the infinite consciousness. A person who achieves such realisation attains eternal bliss, is free from the limitations of time and is released from the cycle of birth-death-rebirth.

Ancient Indian tradition is neither life denying nor otherworldly. Whilst it does not uphold the fulfilment of worldly desires, it acknowledges the necessity of wealth (*artha*) and pleasure (*kama*). However it repeatedly reminds its followers of the transitory and uncertain quality of wealth and pleasure and of their inability to grant lasting satisfaction. It lays emphasis on the third goal – *dharma*. *Dharma* requires us to fulfil our duties towards man and god and to be attentive to the welfare of the whole even as we pursue our individual needs.

An ancient Indian invocation has the physician praying for the welfare of his patients thus:

"May all be at ease."
"May all be sinless."
"May all experience happiness."
"May none experience suffering."

## Medical Ethics in Ancient India

### Philosophy Interwoven Into Ayurveda

Philosophy formed the basis of ethical pronouncements in *Ayurveda*.

*Ayur* defines the purpose of classical Indian medicine as the *prolongation and preservation of life*. *Veda* anchors the science within the Hindu religious tradition. Ayurveda was a secondary science (*upanga*) linked to the *Atharva Veda*.

Above all, *Ayurveda* aims at the attainment of salvation by which the human mind realises the identity of the individual soul with the universal consciousness and thus rises above unhappiness, pain and mortal destruction. *The goal of ayurveda is the cultivation of a sound mind in a healthy body as a means towards ensuring the welfare of the soul and ending the cycle of rebirths.*

Zimmer has summed it up well: "Ayurveda carefully gathered and sifted the rich inheritance from the preceding generations and inter-related the philosophic background of medicine with religious thought, spiritual life and ideals."

### Some Ethical Declarations

*Qualities required in a student.* Not all persons are fit to be students of medicine. Acceptance or rejection of pupils was left to the ancient Indian preceptor. The preceptor, who has set his mind on teaching, should first examine the person who presents himself as a pupil, to see that he possesses certain physical, moral and intellectual endowments.

*Caraka* and *Susruta* listed the following requirements of the student:

- Noble by nature, devoted to truth, intelligent, of a thoughtful disposition, courageous, compassionate;
- Excellent character; pure in his behaviour; devoted, clever and compassionate to all;
- Endowed with broad understanding, power of judgement and memory, liberal mind;
- Disposed to solitude, fond of study, devotedly attached to both the theory and practice of medicine;
- Self-control;
- Seeks the good of all creatures;
- Free from haughtiness, pride, wrath, cupidity, sloth;
- Free from those faults which are grouped under the *vyasanas* – hunting; gambling with dice; sleeping during the day; speaking ill of others; infatuation with women; addiction to singing, dancing and instrumental music; purposeless sauntering....

*Qualities required in a teacher.* Not all persons can become teachers.

*Caraka* and *Susruta* listed the following requirements of the teacher:

- Compassionate towards those who approach him;
- Pure of conduct;
- Clever, experienced, well-disposed towards disciples and disposed to teach them;
- Without malice or a wrathful disposition;
- Capable of bearing privations and pain;
- Capable of communicating his ideas to pupils seeking his instructions;
- Knowledge of the medical sciences has been supplemented by knowledge of other branches of study;
- Conversant with the nature of health, disease, medicaments, time, place, men;
- Conversant with the tendencies and acts of the healthy and of the diseased;
- Possesses all the organs of sense;
- Possesses all the implements of his profession;
- A practised hand.

## Duties of the Teacher

Two principal duties were emphasised:

- Imparting detailed knowledge of the various branches and regions of the science of life.
- Explaining its philosophical basis and the real sig-

nificance of the diverse information found in the various authoritative texts.

The student was not to be made to limit his studies to *Ayurveda* alone but was to include as much as possible of all other branches of science and philosophy which must be known for a true understanding of the human being.

The student was made to understand that the formal training is only the minimum equipment of the physician. It is only after adequate experience through years of practice, observations, further study and discussions that a person can aspire to be worthy of the profession.

If he failed to keep up this schedule of constant improvement, he was to be regarded not as a true physician but merely as an impostor.

## Instructions to the Disciple at the Consecration Ceremony.

- It is the duty of all good physicians to treat gratuitously with their own medicines, all Brahmins, spiritual guides, paupers, friends, ascetics, neighbours, devotees, orphans and people who come from a distance as if they are his own friends.
- If you desire to achieve success of treatment and win heaven hereafter, you should always seek, whether standing or sitting, the good of all living creatures.
- You should, with your whole heart, strive to bring about the cure of those that are ill.
- You should speak words that are soft, unstained by impurity, full of righteousness, incapable of giving pain to others, truthful, beneficial and properly weighed and measured.
- Even if possessed of sufficient knowledge, you should not boast of that knowledge.
- You should always strive to acquire knowledge, cast off sloth, keep ready the implements and medicines you may require.
- You should give up lust, anger, avarice, folly, vanity, pride, envy, rudeness, deception, falsehood, idleness and all other reprehensible conduct.
- You should not, even in imagination, know another man's wife.
- You should not appropriate other people's possessions.
- Whilst entering the family dwelling-place of the patient, you should do it after giving notice to the inmates and with their permission. Some male member of the family should accompany you. You

should cover your person properly. You should keep your face downwards. With your wits about you, you should, with understanding and mind properly focussed, observe all things. Having entered, you should not devote your words, mind, understanding and senses on anything else than what is calculated to do good to the patient or to any other object connected with the patient than his recovery.
- You should never give out to others the practices of the patient's home.
- Even if you be certain of it, you should not speak of the diminution of the period of the patient's life when such speaking may shock the patient or anybody else.
- There is no end to medical science, hence, heedfully devote yourself to it.

## Some Aphorisms for the Student

- Learning by rote, without understanding the meaning of what is thus committed to memory is like an ass carrying a load of sandalwood, and is labour without profit. As the ass which carries the load perceives the weight but not the fragrance of sandalwood, so the dunces who study numerous *sastras* (learned works) without understanding their meaning.
- After studying the *sastras* the art of healing has to be learned practically... Without practical training, repeated recitation or hearing of lessons will not qualify the pupil for practice... He who is only trained in theory but not experienced in practice knows not what to do when he has a patient and behaves as foolishly as a youth upon a battlefield. On the other hand, a physician who is educated practically, but not in theory, will not earn the respect of better men.
- Unto men possessed of intelligence, the entire world acts as a preceptor. Unto men destitute of intelligence, the world occupies the position of enemy. Hence, observing all this, an intelligent man should listen and act up to the counsels of the one who is even a foe when these happen to be instructive and praiseworthy.
- The physician conversant with his science, reflecting in all manner of ways, upon everything, as far as is possible, should then come to a conclusion about the diagnosis of the disease before him and the treatment that should be followed.

- The physician of knowledge, who fails to enter the inner body of the patient with the lamp of knowledge and understanding, can never treat diseases.
- Patients trust their physicians implicitly to the extent of placing their lives unhesitatingly under his care. This is true even of patients who have no trust in their own relations, parents and sons. Hence a physician should take as much care of each and every patient as he would of his own family.
- By following these principles, the physician benefits his fellow-creatures, achieves glory and merit in this world and creates a place for himself in heaven after death.

## The First Medical Conference Ever

Learning at meetings and conferences has always been encouraged in Indian medicine. The first medical conference, ever, in India, is part of legend and appears to have taken place in those ancient times when men and gods intermixed.

The origins of Indian medicine have been traced to a critical stage when moral perfection and saintliness, prevalent from the ideal beginnings of time, decreased; disease made its appearance and the span of life was shortened. The fulfilment of religious duties became impossible.

Out of compassion for mankind, the sages gathered on an auspicious slope of the Himalayas and meditated on the problem; holding, in the process, what may have been the first medical seminar ever. The theme: "By what means can disease be checked, since freedom from disease is the elementary requirement for all religious, secular and spiritual pursuits?"

As a result of the supplications made by this group, their leader, *Bharadvaja*, was received by *Indra* at his celestial abode. *Indra* then revealed *Ayurveda* to him. *Bharadvaja* grasped the knowledge on the causes of disease, symptoms and remedies and brought it back to earth to pass it on to the assembled wise men who, in turn, incorporated it into the various *Samhitas* which have been handed down to us.

## Relationships Between Doctors

*Caraka* advised physicians to hold discussions with their colleagues. Discussion increases the zeal for knowledge, clarifies understanding, increases the power of speech, removes doubts and strengthens convictions. In the course of these discussions, many new things can be learnt.

These discussions are of two types: friendly or hostile. A friendly discussion is held between wise and learned persons who frankly and sincerely discuss questions and give their views without any fear of being defeated or of the fallacies of their arguments being exposed in such discussions. Even though fallacies may be voiced, no one tries to take advantage of the other, no one is jubilant over the other's defeat and no attempt is made to misinterpret the other's views.

*Caraka Samhita* provides hints on how a good and clever physician can defeat his opponents in hostile dispute, by sophisticated wrangling and the use of tricks of logic. This was taught because it was often necessary for these physicians to earn their bread in the face of strong competition.

## The Ethics of the Profession

A passage in the *Caraka Samhita* summed up the ethical injunctions of that time:

"He who practices medicine out of compassion for all creatures rather than for gain or for gratification of the senses surpasses all."

"Those who for the sake of making a living make a trade of medicine, bargain for a dust-heap, letting go a heap of gold."

"No benefactor, moral or material, compares to the physician who by severing the noose of death in the form of fierce diseases, brings back to life those being dragged towards death's abode, because there is no other gift greater than the gift of life."

"He who practices medicine while holding compassion for all creatures as the highest religion is a man who has fulfilled his mission. He obtains supreme happiness."

## Quacks

*Caraka* speaks of them as 'cheats who wander about on the streets boasting in the garb of physicians.'

"As soon as they hear of a patient, they hurry there and boast loudly of their medical capacities so as to reach his ears. They try to win over his friends by all sorts of attentions and emphasise that they would be satisfied with small remuneration. When they treat a patient and cannot allay his pain, they assert that he did not take the necessary remedies, disobeyed their directions and could not control his desires."

"When the case is hopeless, they run away. They

boast of their skill before uneducated people and, by doing so, only betray their ignorance. They avoid assemblies of learned people just as a traveller avoids a dangerous forest. Nobody knows of their teacher, pupil or fellow-pupil. Such quacks are particularly responsible for the bad reputation of physicians."

## Ancient Thoughts on Current Ethical Dilemmas

We encounter a dilemma when values to which we are equally committed are brought into conflict, so that the honouring of one value necessitates the violation of the other.

The ancient Indian position is to be distinguished from that of the religious fundamentalist who views dilemmas in the light of revelation; and that of the secular rationalist, who views them as problems to be solved by reason. For the one the problem is the need for better faith; for the other it is the need for superior knowledge. In either case, there are no genuine dilemmas.

Indian ethics acknowledges genuine moral dilemmas. Examples of apparently irreconcilable alternatives abound in the epic literature.

The *Bhagvadgita* opens with a dilemma tugging at the heart and mind of *Arjuna*, as this lonesome warrior faces the choice of having to kill or be killed by his own kinsmen.

### Can an Ethical Principle Ever be Broken?

*Arjuna* had promised *Agni*, the fire God, that he would kill anyone who spoke ill of his *Gandiva* bow. When his elder brother *Yudhisthira* insulted *Arjun* and his *Gandiva* bow on the very day of the final encounter, he felt that he would now either have to kill his elder brother or break his promise.

*Krsna*, however, argued thus with *Arjuna*: Promise-keeping or even truth-telling cannot be an unconditional obligation when it is in conflict with the avoidance of grossly unjust and criminal acts such as patricide or fratricide. Saving the innocent life of his elder brother is also a strong obligation. Hence, according to *Krsna*, two almost equally strong obligations or duties are in conflict here.

*Krsna* then argued that the *dharmic* thing to do is to be guided by the demands of the situation. There is no question about the need to maintain the consistency of an ethical system, but sometimes the infraction of these values is permitted to achieve nobler ends. This does

not reduce ethics to opportunism; but neither is it made the captive of absolutism.

The point is also illustrated by *Krsna's* story about *Kausika*, a hermit who had taken a vow always to speak the truth. One day, while seated at the crossroad, this holy man was begged by a band of fleeing travellers not to divulge their escape route to bandits who pursued them with the intention of taking their lives. *Kausika* did not reply. When the bandits arrived at the scene, knowing full well that the hermit would not tell a lie, they asked about the travellers and *Kausika* told them the truth. The travellers were caught and killed. *Kausika's* fate was equally sad. Though he had faithfully practised virtue in order to reach heaven, he failed to achieve his goal because, in this instance, truth telling was a violent act which emptied his store of merit.

Clearly, the demand of the situation was the overriding duty to save precious lives, even though to effect this meant telling a lie. But *Kausika* was an absolutist who could not see that telling the truth ceased being an unconditional obligation when weighed in the balance against the need for preserving lives.

This lesson can serve as a guide when we worry about how much we should tell the patient.

The internal flexibility of Hindu ethics gives it a certain advantage over two current social positions on life-and-death issues – *authoritarianism* and *relativism* – by the importance it gives to rational authority. Whilst Hinduism recognises revelation, it does not depreciate the role of reason.

### Abortion

Classic Indian medical manuals place the highest premium on life in general, including that within the womb. Foeticide is murder. Pregnant women are subjects of solicitude and are treated with kindness and care. Abortion is a morally reprehensible killing (*hatya*), bearing the greatest guilt. In a pyramid of evil, it is classified as one of the most atrocious acts.

At the same time, Hinduism states that the right to life of the foetus is not absolute. It addresses competing rights and values. Ethical dilemmas arise in the case of rape and incest and when the mother runs the risk of grave injury or death from continued pregnancy. The physician is asked to keep the interests of the mother uppermost.

Where the mother's life is in a balance, Hindu ethics places greater weight on maternal right to life than that of the foetus. A rational explanation is offered for this choice. The mother has arrived at a *karmic* state in which there is much more at stake for her spiritual destiny. She has obligations to be performed for her family and society. This is why she must be favoured over an equal human being whose evolution in life is, by comparison, rudimentary and who has not yet established a social network of relationships and responsibilities.

With abortion as with euthanasia, the quality that Hinduism calls upon in tragic situations is *daya* or compassion.

### Death

Death is not the opposite of life but the opposite of birth. The expectation of numerous rebirths diminishes the tragedy of death for the Hindu.

Life and death are points on a continuum. Death is the separation of the *atman* or soul from the physical body. In the case of one who has not achieved *moksha*, the *atman*, consistent with its own *karma* will find another appropriate physical body.

The *Brhadaranyaka Upanisad* likens death in old age to the separation of a ripe fruit from its stalk and emphasises that it is not to be seen as an abnormal feature of human existence.

"When this [body] becomes thin – is emaciated through old age or disease – then, as a mango or a fig or a fruit of the *peepul* tree is detached from its stalk, so does this infinite being, completely detaching himself from the spare parts of the body, again go, in the same way that he came, to particular bodies, for the unfoldment of his vital force."

In the vision of the *Upanisads*, for the individual who has come to understand the identity of the self (*atman*) with the ultimate reality of all things (*Brahman*) there is no departure. At the time of physical death, the body disintegrates into its constituent elements and the *atman*, free from all egocentric characteristics that perpetuate its individuality, merges into the subtle elements. The self, transcending all dualities of space and time, abides as itself. Liberated from life whilst within the body (*jivan mukti*), such a person is liberated in death without the body (*videha mukti*). 'Being *Brahman*, he is merged in *Brahman*.'

### Assisted Suicide, Euthanasia

The reverence Hindu philosophy holds for life leads it to advocate the protection and preservation of life in all circumstances. As such, it condemns all acts that destroy life.

At the same time, Hindu ethics displays a certain tolerance and flexibility in the context of individual intentions, motives and circumstances.

There is support for the right to suicide on the grounds of autonomy and rational choice, but this is only a limited right – a religious option permitted in the pursuit of higher goals. Euthanasia is acceptable under the Hindu tradition only on religious grounds.

*Assisted suicide* on religious grounds is not frowned upon, the authorised *modus operandi* for such an act including immolation, drowning, poisoning, falling and fasting.

*Active euthanasia* – the intentional ending of the life of a terminally ill or dying person who is enduring intractable pain and who wishes a merciful end of life – is permitted under Hindu philosophy. The basis for this sanction is as follows:

- Tradition states that only activity arising from selfish motives produce *karma*. Disinterested actions are not only free of ill consequences but can help dissipate the *karma* of our past and present life which has not yet begun to bear fruit. Thus, there is room for action which can undo the ill effects of both past and the present *karma*. With the proper motives, man has it in his power to turn back the past and transform the future.
- Since God dwells in all beings, to help those in distress is to help God. To fail to come to the aid of a sufferer would be to incur sin, for one would thereby be refusing to serve God – who is immanent in that suffering being.

In keeping with the ancient tradition, which allowed an enlightened person to choose the precise time of his death, it is morally permissible for him to do so with medical aid should he find himself terminally ill or in great pain. He knows that his mind can control his body today. In a short while, his body will control his mind. Excruciating suffering will then rob him of the equanimity he so cherishes for his final moments of life. Euthanasia ensures a merciful death because he can leave this life with consciousness unclouded by the stupor of drugs.

One who has lived a long and fruitful life is more concerned about the quality of life than the inevitability of death. That especially applies to life's end. A 'good death' is a spiritual death. The individual is in a psychologically balanced state of mind, composed and in control. His heart and heart are free – without the wish either to live or to die. To ensure such a death, Hindu ethics permits the purposive shortening of a person's life.

Hinduism emphasises that *living* is more important than *being alive*. This places Hinduism squarely on the side of those who would argue for active euthanasia on the grounds of the quality of life over the claims of purposeless existence.

*The argument of the Golden Rule.* Hinduism's strong sense of the sacredness of life expresses itself in diverse forms, including the Golden Rule. There are various instances in the epic literature. The *Mahabharata* first exhorts the norm of self-similitude: "Good people do not injure living beings; in joy and sorrow, pleasure and pain, one should act towards others as one would have them act toward oneself." And then, more broadly: "Whatever one would wish for oneself, that let one plan for another."

Hindu ethics cherishes the principle of *daya* or compassion, mythologically personified as a daughter of *Daksha* and the wife of *Dharma*. If we want the rule of euthanasia, in dire circumstances, to apply to us, then it follows that we must want the same rule to apply to others.

Hindu ethics rules out *involuntary euthanasia* as this involves the taking the life of an individual, supposedly in his own interests, but either against his own wishes or without the benefit of consultation. It flatly contradicts the principle of autonomy and is fraught with ominous side effects.

*Passive euthanasia* is often identified with the stopping of treatment that is no longer beneficial to the patient. As long as the individual has a fighting chance of regaining health, Hindu ethics would acknowledge the obligation to preserve life, but where such prospects have vanished, that obligation disappears.

The classic example of such a death is provided in the *Mahabharata*. "The heroic *Bhishma* turned to *Duryodhana*, the king, and said, 'Give generous and befitting presents of money to these good surgeons and pay them due honour and send them away, for *to me in this condition no treatment is welcome... I must be allowed to die ...*'"

*Ayurvedic* medicine recognises that there are limits to our responsibility to preserve life. The injunction 'Do not resuscitate' was applied in ancient India (as, indeed, in ancient Greece) to diseases that were deemed incurable. Caraka commented: "The physi-cian treating an incurable disease certainly suffers from the loss of wealth, learning and reputation and from censure and unpopularity... A wise physician should ... take up the treatment only in case of curable diseases."

*Caraka* advised withholding medications from a dying patient but allowed nutrition should the family insist on it.

Hindu ethics disallows the killing of an individual incapable of formulating a preference or being able to communicate it.

Summing up, Hindus renounce all forms of killing and *ahimsa* serves as a general guide. At the same time the pro-life principle in Hinduism is not absolute. Hindu ethics is not passive in the face of suffering. We are not given the right to keep terminally ill people alive and in pain when all they want is a peaceful death. Their *karma* is our *dharma*. We have a duty to our fellow-beings. If they are suffering because of some sin, it is no less a sin to let them suffer.

*Suicide and the Right to Die*

Whilst a vibrant 'will to life' is reiterated in numerous *Vedic* prayers, longevity is not simply valued in terms of duration, but by the quality of life – which should remain full of vitality and virtue. The *Atharva Veda* illustrates this:

"For a hundred autumns, may we see,
For a hundred autumns, may we live,
For a hundred autumns, may we know ...
For a hundred autumns, may we thrive ...
Aye, and even more than a hundred autumns."

Another section prays: "May all my limbs be uninjured and my soul remain unconquered."

Suicide was viewed in the light of man's duties. Each one of us has threefold obligations – duty to the gods through sacrifice; obligation to perpetuate the family and uphold cultural heritage. Death before these obligations have been met would lead to rebirth. This sense of social obligation is a powerful deterrent against the idea of taking one's one life.

Ancient Indians classified the stages of life into four *asramas*:

*Brahmacarya* – celibacy, study and gaining of experience;
*Grhasthya* – forming and sustaining a household;
*Vanaprasthya* – detachment from worldly affairs,

emigration to a secluded place such as the forest for contemplation;

*Sanyasa* – life as a hermit, spiritual quest to understand the ultimate consciousness, preparation for death.

The sage prays

From the unreal (*asat*) lead me to the real (*sat*)!
From darkness lead me to light!
From death lead me to immortality!

This philosophy necessitated changes in needs and aspirations over time. Inevitably, values placed on life and death too altered.

The *Vedas* and *Upanisads* taught that everyday existence is insignificant compared with the experience of mystical union, which carries one beyond this ephemeral world. In later works such as the *Jabala* and *Kanthasruti Upanisads*, the enlightened *sanyasin* is instructed to choose voluntary death in some heroic manner.

The practice of religious suicide has a very respectable antiquity in India. Megasthenes of Kalanos, the Indian gymnosophist from Taxila who had accompanied Alexander the Great from India provided an example. At the age of 73, he burnt himself alive on a funeral pyre at Sousa, being 'afflicted with a malady that made life more and more burdensome.' This incident took place in the 4th century B.C. but it is probable that the practice of religious suicide was in vogue long before that time. Not only was there an absence of guilt but there was a sense of acquisition of merit.

The goal of complete union with the supreme Soul, extreme bodily hardships and immersion in the sacred texts made suicide appear a natural end. Society sanctioned such a step.

*Manu* points out the path to be followed by one intending to end his life:

"He should sleep on raised ground and should feel no concern if he suffers from an illness. He should neither welcome death nor feel joy for continuing to live, but he should patiently wait till the time of death, as a servant waits till the time he is hired expires."

After describing the conventional path to final liberation, *Manu* adds: "Or let him walk, fully determined and going straight on, in a north-easterly direction, subsisting on water and air, until his body sinks to rest. A person, having got rid of his body by one of those modes practised by the great sages, is exalted in the world of *Brahman*, free from sorrow and fear."

This came to be known as the Great Journey (*mahaprasthana*). Taking the lead from *Manu* and *Yajnavalkya*, other authors recommend a more precipitous option with the exhortation that 'a forest hermit may resort to the distant journey or may enter water or fire or may throw himself from a precipice."

Society also sanctioned another form of suicide. The criminal, condemned to death, was given the option to commit suicide as a penitential act that would secure expiation of his offences.

There were many other reasons for which people killed themselves. Some felt that life no longer held any purpose. They had lived their lives upholding moral principles, but now that type of life no longer had any appeal and they longed for release from the weary cycle of birth and death. If the burden of old age or the bane of disease were added to this feeling, they wished quickly to put an end to it all. Suicide by drowning was commended, especially at an auspicious place such as Prayaga, where the holy *Ganga* and *Yamuna* come together with the invisible *Saraswati*. To drown oneself at the *sangama* is to enter *moksha*, which is ordinarily open only to the yogi who achieves this end through a lifetime of discipline and learning.

A more benign though highly meritorious form of suicide was through fasting. The *Anusasanaparva* of the *Mahabharata* claims: "A man, who, knowing the Vedanta and understanding the ephemeral nature of life abandons life in the Himalayas by fasting, would reach the world of *Brahma*." This method became popular among the Jains. Chandragupta Maurya is the most famous of those who ended their lives through starvation.

To sum up, the Hindu view on suicide has a core and a periphery. The philosophic goal of the centre is the attainment of the highest human value, namely, liberation from *samsara* or the round of rebirths. The moral values which facilitate this goal are those which preserve and promote a quality of life commensurate with spiritual aspiration.

Within this philosophic framework, Hinduism condemns suicide as evil when it is a direct and deliberate act with the intention voluntarily to kill oneself for self-serving motives. Such suicide is a product of ignorance and passion. It also has negative *karmic* consequences impeding *moksha*.

Hinduism permits religiously motivated suicide by one who has attained *sanyasa* – the fourth and final stage of life.

We must look upon the world as home and not be

overanxious, even for dire reasons to make a hasty exit. On the other hand, should we reach the point when, through disability, age or disease the body is no longer capable of keeping pace with the spirit, then the body may respectfully be left behind.

Suicide brings about death. Whilst there is an end to the physical body, individuality of the self persists. The latter is ends only when, after enlightenment, the individual realises union with the Supreme Reality.

While affirming the cardinal principle of sanctity of life, Hinduism allows the right to suicide on the basis of rational choice and personal autonomy.

There is a respectful acceptance of an individual's wish for a peaceful and ennobling death, having renounced all earthly attachments and all desires, including desires for the avoidance of suffering and the hope of happiness in some future existence.

Because this state of mind and spirit is possible only for the few who have led a disciplined life, it is assumed that the person who is fully capable for making this awesome decision must be a sage or an ascetic. For such a perfect one, suicide is eternal release from the wheel of rebirth (samsara) and awakening of the soul.

## Brain Death and Organ Transplantation

The *Vedas* pointed out that the brain was the most important organ in the human body. It was the residence of the mind and governed all our senses. When the brain is destroyed, there is loss of consciousness, cessation of breathing, paralysis of limbs and death. The association of loss of consciousness, paralysis of breathing and death appears to anticipate the current concept of brain death following irreparable damage to the brain stem.

Ancient Indian scriptures contain an account of what could be considered the first organ transplant ever – the implantation of the head of an elephant on to the trunk of *Ganesha*, the son of Lord *Siva*.

The ethical principles that govern the care of the sick and advocate doing everything possible to cure illness and preserve life apply to organ transplantation. As long as such an operation is carried out with the noblest of intentions and without wilful harm to any other, Hindu philosophy and ethics sanctions it.

Removal of organs from an individual deemed to be brain dead is in keeping with ancient Indian ethics. Since the body is a mere vehicle for the *atman*, it can be dealt with in any manner deemed suitable by society once the *atman* had departed from it. The ancient Indian sage would have no difficulty in permitting the use of organs from a dead individual for the benefit of sick persons.

The rampant malpractice witnessed in modern India where organs are bought and sold or stolen after misrepresentation of facts is evidently immoral and unethical.

## Medical Ethics in India Today

### Introduction

Doctors are not made to face ethical dilemmas during their medical training.

Indian doctors, schooled in Western science, are ignorant of the medical ethics of their own culture. A conscious effort is made by them to distance themselves from *Ayurvedic* medicine, in which the ethical codes are enshrined. Teachers and students forget that values have universal applicability, regardless of the mode of practice – Western or traditional – and that the patient remains the same regardless of the system.

The *Caraka* and *Susruta Samhitas* are a rich repository of ethical codes pertaining to the training, duties and privileges of the physician. The desire for success, wealth and fame on the part of the doctor are deemed proper and normal, provided ambition is balanced by meeting obligations to patients and to society.

As we examine the tangled state of Indian medical ethics, we are increasingly aware that wide sections of our ethical roofing are perched perilously. Nowhere is this crisis more pressing than in respect to issues of life and death. As we survey the scene, we find a widespread sense of moral disarray. We've had a traditional set of standards which have been disregarded and are no longer fashionable. We have lost our moral landmarks. With the breakdown of the traditional consensus, there is no more debate. The scarcity of role models for the medical neophyte only aggravates the malady.

### A Poor Start

Unethical practices in getting entry into medical colleges as students are rampant. Private medical colleges necessitate huge capital investments by each medical student. On graduation, there is a need to recover these investments and generate profit on them as soon as the doctor starts practice.

## Lack of Teaching

There is but one institution in India (St. John's Medical College, Bangalore) that offers a structured course on medical ethics throughout the undergraduate curriculum.

In almost all other teaching institutions, medical ethics is dealt with cursorily, if at all. There are no sessions where real life dilemmas are highlighted and the principles to be invoked in solving them discussed.

Under these circumstances it is not surprising that students emerging from almost all our medical colleges are ill-equipped to ask questions of themselves or ponder the nature and consequences of their own actions towards patients and their families.

## Absence of Role Models

Rampant profiteering by senior and established medical consultants and family physicians worsens the situation. Getting rich quickly by any means is the norm.

The impressionable student sees his teachers ill-treat and cheat his patients, extort large sums illegally and do everything possible to deprive the government of taxes due on their incomes. Such observations encourage the student – already under family and societal pressure to make good rapidly – to follow suit. Over the past five decades or so, we have one generation influencing another in unethical practices to result in the present appalling situation.

## Inroads Made by Commercialism

The spirit of privatisation now pervades India. Whilst the benefits have been widely publicised, the drawbacks have been little discussed.

Hitherto, poor patients had free access to the best that the medical sciences had to offer at the public hospitals run by governments (central and state) and municipal corporations. These hospitals were created for the poor patient and the costs were wholly subsidised.

Rising costs and the wave of privatisation have combined to throw these hospitals to the winds. Administrators and bureaucrats now seek ways to raise income from the abjectly poor patients who throng their institutions. When such funds cannot be raised, the hospitals are allowed to decay and disintegrate. In my own city, Mumbai, we are now witnesses to a public hospital being auctioned to the highest bidder.

Commercialism has had other ill consequences. Let me give you some examples.

Smelling fast bucks, several individuals (some of them medical consultants themselves) or groups, have set up Computerised Tomography and Magnetic Resonance scanners in most major cities. The intense competition between these centres has engendered the pernicious system of fee splitting. The doctor referring a patient for a scan is paid a handsome fee for 'prescan clinical workup'! Unscrupulous clinicians – and there are plenty of them – have been quick to seize this opportunity and refer every patient with a headache or a backache for such scans, often without a detailed clinical examination. It is particularly regrettable that some members of the Neurological Society of India are party to such practices since one of the first goals of this Society at its foundation was 'to maintain the highest ethical standards in the practice of this speciality'.

The advent of corporate hospitals set up purely with a motive to make huge profits and offer dividends to their shareholders has aggravated the sharp departure from ethical practice. Chains of hospitals are being set up with a holding company, a subsidiary for making centralised purchases for the entire chain, and individual companies for each hospital. The holding company often ensures that equipment is purchased from predetermined firms, often for considerations other than merit. Channelling all purchases through a centralised subsidiary ensures fat returns on each item purchased for the entire chain. In the process, the patient pays hugely inflated costs.

## Journal on Medical Ethics

We have but one journal on medical ethics in India. Even this is floundering for want of support. The secretary of the Department of Biotechnology, Government of India promised financial support to the journal in an open, international meeting. This promise has not been honoured. Medical ethics has zero priority in the minds of administrators, teachers and students.

## A General Lack of Character

When the subject of medical ethics is brought up for discussion at meetings of medical doctors, inevitably, someone raises an apparently logical question: "When society at large is corrupt and unethical, how can you expect doctors to remain honest?"

The question assumes that if everyone is doing wrong, we are entitled to follow suit. It also shows that most of us, in the Indian medical profession, though literate are not educated enough to be able to transcend our baser impulses. In doing so, of course, we 'bargain for a dust-heap, letting go a heap of gold'.

We have also forgotten two lessons taught in recent times.

The mystic sage from Bengal, *Ramakrishna Paramhansa* (1836–1886), commented on the Indian penchant for idol worship and offered a suggestion that could be used by all Indian doctors to the advantage of their patients:

"If God can be worshipped in images of clay, should He not be worshipped in one's fellow beings?"

Mahatma Gandhi (1869–1948) offered a talisman to be used when we are in doubt as to the course of an action or when we are obsessed with ourselves and our own wellbeing:

"Recall the face of the poorest and weakest man whom you may have seen and ask yourself if the step you contemplate is going to be of use to him... Then you will find your doubt and yourself melting away ..."

## Glossary

| | |
|---|---|
| *Ahimsa* | Non-violence |
| *Artha* | Wealth |
| *Asramas* | Stages of life |
| *Atman* | Soul |
| *Ayurveda* | From *Ayur* – life, and *veda* – divine knowledge. The science of life. |
| *Brahma* | One of the three members of the Hindu Pantheon. Known as the Creator. |
| *Brahman* | The eternal, all-pervading consciousness. God. (Note: The highest caste amongst the Hindus is also named the Brahman community.) |
| *Bhagvadgita* | Hindu epic. Part of the *Mahabharata*. A treasury of ancient Indian philosophy. |
| *Caraka* | Ancient Indian physician. Author of *Caraka Samhita*. |
| *Daya* | Compassion |
| *Dharma* | Duties, obligations and responsibilities. |
| *Jivan Mukti* | Freedom of the soul from rebirth |
| *Kama* | Pleasure |
| *Karma* | A record of thoughts and actions that will determine the manner and form of rebirth. |
| *Mahabharata* | Hindu epic. It incorporates the *Bhagvadgita*. |
| *Mahaprasthana* | The Great Journey – from life to death |
| *Manu* | An ancient law-giver |
| *Moksha* | Liberation. Freedom of the soul from the cycle of life-birth-life. |
| *Peepul* | The fig tree |
| *Prayaga* | Near Allahabad in the northern Indian state of Uttar Pradesh where the rivers *Ganga* and *Jamuna* join the mythical river *Saraswati* |
| *Samhita* | Medical text |
| *Samsara* | Life on earth – part of the cycle of life-death-rebirth |
| *Sangama* | Union – as that of three rivers at *Prayaga* |
| *Sanyasin* | One who has renounced material life and given himself up to spiritual quest |
| *Sastras* | Learned texts |
| *Susruta* | Ancient Indian surgeon. Author of *Susruta Samhita* |
| *Upanisad* | Supplement to the *Veda*, at times incorporating commentaries |
| *Veda* | Hallowed ancient religious and philosophical revelations by the gods. There are four principal *Vedas: Rg, Sam, Yajur* and *Atharva*. |
| *Videha mukti* | Freedom of the soul from death |
| *Vyasanas* | Vices |

## Acknowledgements

I am deeply obliged to Professor Dr. H. A. M. Alphen and his team for the invitation to prepare this paper and for making it possible for me to attend the 9th Convention of the Academia Eurasiana Neurochirurgica.

I have borrowed heavily from the texts referred to below and from other texts not easily available outside India. I have also benefited from discussions with several of my colleagues.

Mr. Chandrakant Shah and Mr. Satish Kulkarni has been of immense help in collecting material for this essay. Mr. Kulkarni also provided the slides used at the presentation at the Convention.

## Suggested Reading

(Note: I have only provided references to texts easily available to the Western reader.)

## References

1. Bhagavat Sinh Jee: Aryan medical science: a short history. Rare Reprints 1981, Delhi
2. Chattopadhyaya Debiprasad (1977) Science and society in ancient India. Research India Publication, Calcutta
3. Chattopadhyaya Debiprasad (ed) Studies in the history of science of India, vol. 1. Editorial Enterprises, (year of publication not mentioned), New Delhi
4. Coward Harold (ed) (1997) Life after death in world religions. Sir Garib Das Oriental Series No. 238. Sri Satguru Publications (a division of Indian Books Centre) (Original publisher: Maryknoll, NY, Orbis Books), Delhi
5. Cromwell Crawford S (1997) Dilemmas of life and death. Hindu ethics in North American context. Sri Satguru Publications, Delhi
6. Filliozat J (1964) The classical doctrine of Indian medicine. Munshiram Manoharlal, Delhi
7. Jolly Julius (1977) Indian medicine. Munshiram Manoharlal, Delhi
8. Kane PV (1973) History of Dharmasastra. Bhandarkar Oriental Institute, Pune
9. Kutumbiah P (1962) Ancient Indian medicine. Orient Longmans, Bombay
10. Mehta PM (ed) (1949) Caraka Samhita. Gulab Kunverba Society, Jamnagar
11. Mukopadhyaya Girindranath (1974) History of Indian medicine. Vol. 1–3. Oriental Books Reprint Corporation, New Delhi
12. Ray P, Gupta HN, Roy M (1980) Susruta Samhita. A scientific synopsis. Indian National Science Academy, New Delhi
13. Svoboda Robert E (1992) Ayurveda. Life, health and longevity. Penguin Books, Arkana
14. Zimmer HR (1948) Hindu medicine. Johns Hopkins Press, Baltimore
15. Zysk Kenneth G (1991) Asceticism and healing in ancient India. Medicine in the Buddhist monastery. Oxford University Press, Delhi
16. Zysk Kenneth G (1996) Medicine in the veda – religious healing in the veda – with translations and annotations of medical hymns from the Rgveda and the Atharvaveda and rendering from the corresponding ritual texts. Motilal Banarsidass Publishers Private Limited, Delhi

Correspondence: Dr. Sunil K. Pandya, Flat 11, 5th floor, Shanti Kutir, Marine Drive, Mumbai 400020, India.

Acta Neurochir (1999) [Suppl] 74: 47–52

# Biblical Moral and Religious Principles in Medical Practice

**R. Evers, Rabbi**

Nederlands Israëlitisch Kerkgenootschap, Amsterdam, The Netherlands.

## Introduction

The Jewish religious and moral directives represent the accumulated wisdom and intellectual labours of millenia, stretching from the Talmud, the codes of Jewish law and their authoritative commentaries, to the most recent rabbinical responsa. All are inspired by the absolute Divine truths enshrined in the Bible, the eternal guide to Jewish conduct. They are founded on the concept of the supreme sanctity of human life and on the dignity of man as a creation in the Image of God.

## The Interface of Medical Ethics and Religion

Judaism does not intrude into the physician's medical prerogatives, provided the considerations in question are purely medical in character. However, modern medicine has moved into new areas in which great moral issues are involved. Organ transplantation, genetic engineering, abortion, contraception, euthanasia, and drug addiction raise serious moral issues. In these areas, Judaism has a message; Judaism has an opinion. The validity of this opinion is confirmed by thousands of years of empirical evidence.

The physician is the expert in the medical evidence. He is the one to provide the medical facts from which a moral judgment must be made. But although, like all men, the physician has a point of view about morals and ethics, this is not his area of special competence.

## The Jewish Definition of Ethical Standards

Judaism, the founding monotheistic religion, embodies within its philosophy and legislation a system of ethics, a definition of moral values. It emphatically insists that the norms of ethical conduct can be governed neither by the accepted notions of public opinion nor by the whims of the individual conscience. Moral values are not matters of subjective choice or personal preference. The human conscience is meant to enforce laws, not to make them. Right or wrong, good and evil are absolute values which transcend the capricious variations of time, place, and environment, as well as human intuition or expediency.

## The Infinite Value of Every Human Life

The first principle in the Jewish approach to medicine is that every human life is of infinite value. From this all-important principle stem numerous practical rulings, such as the suspension of almost all religious laws in the face of any danger to life, the duty to heal the sick as a religious precept, and the prohibition of such acts as suicide, euthanasia and hazardous experimentation on living human beings.

This principle is the indispensable foundation for a moral society. If a person who has only a few minutes or hours more to live would be worth less than one who can still look forward to seventy years of life, the value of every human being would lose its absolute character and become relative, relative to his life expectancy, his state of health, intelligence, his usefulness to society, or any other arbitrary criteria. Such a reduction of human value from absolute to relative, standards would thus vitiate the equality of all men; it would be the thin edge of the wedge dividing mankind into people of superior and inferior value; into those who would have a greater and others who have a lesser claim to life. The moment any human being is toppled from the infinitely high pedestal on which he stands, he drags down with him all others, and the whole fabric of the moral order is bound to collapse.

The slow erosion of the moral ethic is an oft repeated occurrence in the history of many social orders. First the nearly dead are equated with the dead. This value judgment is then extended to encompass the inferior individual. The mentally retarded, the cripple, the unproductive and the undesirable, are then exempted from the guarantee of their inalienable right to life.

## Obstetrics

Judaism regards procreation, and the most intimate of human relations leading to it, as an area of supreme sanctity and privacy. In offering advice and treatment in this delicate area, physicians often face an extraordinary responsibility since their words may determine whether a human being is to be created, to live or die.

In addition to expert medical judgment, such life-and-death decisions require the most competent moral judgment. Such decisions should be taken in consultation with reliable religious guides.

### Abortion

Jewish law sanctions abortions only when continuation of pregnancy is a grave hazard to the mother. Such hazards include psychiatric disturbances which may be caused or aggravated by the continued pregnancy (for example suicidal tendencies). Under such conditions, an abortion must be carried out since the life of the mother is considered to be distinctly superior to that of her unborn child. The fear that a child may be born deformed because the mother contracted Rubella (German measles) or other virus diseases, or took drugs suspected of affecting the child's normal development, does not in itself justify recourse to abortion. Both during and after birth, an abnormal child – whether the defects be mental or physical – enjoys the same title to life as a healthy child. This consideration is quite apart from the chance that an abortion might eliminate a perfectly normal child. The sole indication for terminating a pregnancy under these conditions must therefore be the health of the mother, as previously defined.

### Sterilization.
Surgical or physical impairment of the reproductive organs of any living creature violates Jewish law, except in cases of urgent medical necessity. With males, only a risk to life can justify such procedures. The prohibition against impairing the male reproductive organs and functions is unrelated to man's fertility. It applies even to a man known to have become sterile or impotent, by reason of age or physiological aberration.

During prostatectomy procedures the surgeon should, whenever possible, avoid ligating and cutting the vas deferens. Unless mandated by the disease process, the surgical interruption of any of the structures involved in procreation imposes serious religious problems on the patient – problems that may affect his recovery and future happiness.

### Contraception

Contraceptive devices cannot be used except for halachic (Biblically approved) reasons. Jewish law requires that the marital act be as natural as possible. When medical indications, which include psychological factors, necessitate the use of a contraceptive technique, Jewish law grades these techniques from least to most objectionable in the following order: oral contraceptives, chemical spermicidals, diaphragms and cervical caps to be used by the wife, and condoms. The most objectionable method, and one that is least often sanctioned by Jewish law, is the use by the male of the condom.

Methods which do not interfere with the natural sex act and the normal course of insemination, such as the oral contraceptive pill, would be permitted for lesser reasons – providing their use does not negate the commandment to "be fruitful and multiply".

The "menstrual extraction" technique deserves specific comment. It is more closely associated with the induction of early abortion than are the other methods and hence should not be used except when medically indicated for the welfare of a woman for whom the other contraceptive techniques are contra-indicated.

### Artificial Insemination

The sanctity of the family unit serves as a major tenet of the Jewish faith. The parent-child unit is an essential means of perpetuating the great values of our civilization. Any act that weakens this bond cannot be condoned. It is for this reason that artificial insemination with donor sperm cannot receive routine rabbinic approval. Although the child born of such insemination may not carry the stigma of illegitimacy, in actual practice our religious law discourages this type of insemination.

The main Biblical concern is directed to the secret paternity of the child and the subsequent possibility of incestuous unions between children fathered by the same donor.

## Religion and Psychiatry

The psychiatrist's effort to relieve the patient of incapacitating mental stress is indeed a Biblical commandment. But a note of caution is in order. There is the classic danger of the imposition of the analyst's own value system on that of the patient. If the patient's religious observances, for example, are viewed by the psychiatrist as neurotic or compulsive, rather than as a meaningful life style and a source of stability, the uncritical use of psychiatry can aggravate rather than alleviate the mental stress and be a terrible disservice to the patient.

### Faith Defines Place and Goals in Life

Religion embraces faith and practice. The faith a man lives by, even if undefined, is integral to his personality and defines his place and goals in life. Religious attitudes and practices are emotionally stabilizing, as well as significance-yielding, in their effect. Enforced departure from such routine may create new areas of conflict and guilt. The psychiatrist's attempts to relieve the anxiety should be undertaken with an appreciation of the positive emotional value of the person's religious observance pattern.

### Guilt Feelings

The attitude toward guilt feelings are a fundamental issue of difference between religious and psychiatric counsel. Deep guilt feelings which incapacitate the patient and interfere with his normal functioning are not in consonance with biblical teachings. Because of Judaism's doctrines of repentance and forgiveness, the healthy individual can be loyal to his religious requirements without the adverse effect of morbid guilt feelings. However, guilt feelings concerning willful violations of one's religious, moral or ethical code should not be erased by psychiatric absolution. Instead, the insights of both Judaism and psychiatry ought to be utilized to mitigate the negative effect of guilt feelings, while recognizing that pangs of conscience are necessary goals to human betterment.

### Alienation and Responsibility

The mood of alienation experienced by a growing number of people is best corrected by emphasizing the duties and obligations that characterise man's role in society. The Jewish teaching that joy and fulfillment come from doing what is right may provide a solid basis for therapy. Social functioning and mental health are integrally related to a sense of responsibility.

The complementarity between Judaism and psychiatry is evident. Judaism's emphasis on responsibility, and psychiatry's efforts to restore the impaired sense of capacity for responsibility, can be fruitfully joined.

### Drug Usage

Judaism looks upon drugs as natural agents for the benefit of mankind. However, they are often put to detrimental use as well.

Mood modifying drugs used as an adjunct to medical and ethical counselling can hasten the patient's return to the duties and obligations of the real world. When used uncritically to obliterate anxiety, guilt feelings, or a sense of shame, these drugs short-circuit the ethical early warning signals, subjecting the user to further moral degradation. Discontent is often a necessary prelude to moral and ethical improvement. A mist of alcohol, or marijuana smoke, or the relaxation induced by the much used and abused tranquilizers, can extinguish the soul fire that energises man in his search for self improvement.

The physiological injury these drugs can cause is also of ethical concern. The damage to health that alcoholism or heroin addiction causes, is viewed by Judaism as a matter of religious concern.

## Sexuality

The psychiatrist is usually the key medical counsellor in handling cases involving aberrations in the sexual behaviour of man. Judaism has very clear directives concerning for example sex reversal surgery.

### Sex Reversal Surgery in Adults

Judaism reacts with revulsion to this mutilation, condoned by a small number of surgeons and endocrinologists. It is a violation of Biblical law and of the morals and aesthetics of our society.

*Management of the Newborn with Ambiguous Genitalia*

The determination of a child's sex has many consequences in Jewish law. Maleness incurs special religious obligations. The religious laws prohibiting castration are major considerations in the ethical decision to surgically modify the sex of a newborn.

Current medical practice is to advise the parents to surgically and hormonally convert a biologically male child to a female, when the adult phallus will not be of adequate size or function for sexual relations. Jewish law does not concur with this practice. The consensus of Rabbinic opinion is that surgical castration followed by plastic repair to form the female external genitalia will not cancel out biological and halachic maleness. If such castration was done, the subsequent marriage of the child requires careful Rabbinic consultation.

In true hermaphroditism, or when there is no clearly differentiated gonad, the decision as to the sex identity of the infant must be made after consultation with competent medical and rabbinic authorities.

*Sex Dysfunction*

The sex act is without overtones of guilt or shame in Jewish law when it is performed as an act of love and affection between husband and wife. Dysfunctions of the sex act may seriously weaken the familial bond so essential for our society. Medical and psychiatric advice should be obtained to correct such dysfunctions as impotence, frigidity, premature ejaculation, or insistence on deviant behaviour in the heterosexual relationship. It is regrettable that a byproduct of the so-called sexual revolution is the readiness of the therapist to remove sexual inhibitions in the name of mental health. "Therapeutic adultery", the use of sexual surrogates in therapy, or the violation of other sexual restrictions for this avowed reason cannot be sanctioned by Judaism. These may even violate fundamentals of mental health, aggravating rather than relieving the anxieties of one committed to a moral code.

Skilled counselling in conjunction with Rabbinic consultation to clarify the religious sensitivities of the patient, can often save a marriage in which sex dysfunction is a cause of continual tension and discontent.

## Genetics

What are the ethical implications of this new knowledge? Will it develop into a science designed to "improve and purify the human race" with all the horror that these words impart to civilized men?

*Purpose of Amniocentesis*

When such genetic counselling is sought by a married couple who learned after marriage or after the birth of a deformed child that they are carriers of a genetic defect, they are often advised to resort to foetal monitoring by amniocentesis. This advice is particularly common in the case of the 'Jewish' genetic defect, Tay-Sachs disease. As analysed by Biblical ethics, such amniocentesis is not to be performed if its sole purpose is to determine whether or not to abort the foetus at this stage. The parents must be counselled by Rabbi and physician to assure that they understand the risk incurred by the child (in Tay-Sachs, a 25% chance of contracting the disease and a 50% chance of being a symptom-free carrier) and then to assist them in making their decision to avoid conception by religiously approved means, or to support them in their trust in God's kindness and mercy if they decide to have another child.

*Injurious Knowledge*

Mass screening programs present a special psychological problem. The information they provide can help avoid many tragedies, but this very knowledge may be injurious. The adolescent youth struggling with the psychological stress of his maturation process may be ill equipped to accept with equanimity the knowledge that he is a carrier of a genetic flaw.

*Caring at Home?*

The genetic counsellor is often asked for advice after a deformed or mentally retarded child is born, as to the proper care of this child. Should he be institutionalized or cared for at home? Here too the co-operation of the Rabbi-ethicist can be uniquely helpful. In general, our tradition is to encourage keeping the child within the Jewish family structure unless this be impossible because of the type of care he requires.

## Organ Transplantation

Jewish law is fundamentally opposed to any form of experimentation in which the human organism serves solely as an experimental animal. Even the informed voluntary consent of the participant does not suffice to permit the physician to subject him to hazardous medical procedures.

## Transplantation Surgery and the Indicia of Death

Transplantation surgery presents the problem of the protection of the rights and integrity of the donor. Under Jewish law, imminence of death in no way compromises the inviolable rights and privileges of the donor. One who is in extremis has the full protection of the law; shortening his life by one second is an act of murder. It is therefore categorically prohibited to prepare a critically ill donor for transplantation surgery, if this preparation in any way hastens his death. Donation of an organ is proper only from either a healthy, living patient who has, after careful deliberation with medical and religious authorities, decided to donate a non-vital organ, or from a donor who has already died. Under Jewish law, death is determined by cessation of all respiratory and circulatory activities for a sufficiently long period of time to make resuscitation medically impossible. The current practice of assigning the 'time of death' determination to a team of physicians not involved in the transplantation procedure, is to be commended.

## Care of Patients

### Informing the Patient

In the Jewish view, patients suffering from a fatal illness should not be informed in detail when there is reasonable indication that such knowledge may further impair their physical or mental health. Jewish ethics permit and even require that full facts about the severity of the illness be withheld. The patient should be made aware that he is seriously ill but that there is every expectation that he will be healed. Only in exceptional circumstances may the true facts be communicated to him; the concurrence of physician and rabbi should be obtained. The doctor should never set a "maximum time to live" for any patient. Such estimates are usually destructive of the defense energies of the patient and his family.

### Euthanasia

Judaism condemns any deliberate induction of death, even if the patient so requests, as an act of murder. Life is not ours to terminate. Therefore it is absolutely forbidden to administer any drugs or institute any procedure which may hasten the death of the patient, unless such drugs or procedures have significant therapeutic potential. One of the most perplexing of all medical-moral problems facing the physician is that of passive euthanasia. Judaism does *not* condone either active or passive euthanasia. This term has been used to describe a wide range of morally questionable medical practices.

They include the "near active" euthanasia of prescribing maximal dosages of barbiturates and narcotics with full knowledge that these dosages will physiologically compromise the patient, as well as the withholding of antibiotics so that "the old man's best friend", bronchopneumonia, can bring to a more speedy end the ebbing life force.

The birth of a deformed child in need of life-saving surgery is a problem in passive euthanasia of frequent concern to paediatric surgeons. Should the consummate skill of the surgeon be used to preserve a life of dubious quality?

Centuries of active ethical concern have set the guidelines for a "domino theory" of social ethics. When one seemingly innocuous inroad is made into the inviolate sanctuary of human life, the whole ethical structure of society is threatened with collapse.

The general attitude of Jewish ethics toward medical euthanasia, passive or active, must be clearly understood. The physician has but one commitment to his patient – to prolong his life and to cure him of his illness. Acting in any other capacity, he forfeits the rights and privileges of a physician and must be judged as any other layman who has decided to hasten the death of a critically ill or deformed patient. Thus, active euthanasie is unadorned killing that runs counter to our great philosophical and ethical premises as to the value of residual life.

## Research on Animals

Jewish law sanctions medical research on animals, including vivisection. Unlike our fellow human beings animals are in man's service. It is intellectually dishonest to serve meat at the table and then to lobby for legislation against medical experimentation on animals. However, it is a violation of Biblical law to cause unnecessary pain to animals. During research experiments, every precaution must be taken to protect the animal from unnecessary suffering. Experiments designed to promote human health are in keeping with the religious rules goveming man's relations with infra-human species.

Correspondence: Raphael Evers, LL. M., Rabbi, Nederlands Israëlitisch Kerkgenootschap, Van der Boechorststraat 26, 1081 BT Amsterdam, The Netherlands.

Acta Neurochir (1999) [Suppl] 74: 53–58

# Carrying on the Healing Mission of Christ: Medical Ethics in the Christian Tradition

**W. J. Eijk**, Priest

Faculty of Theology, Lugano, Switzerland.

Speaking of the traditional Christian approach of medical ethics, we should be aware of the fact that, though Christianity has existed for nearly two millennia, medical ethics as a distinct discipline dates from the late Middle Ages and the Renaissance. Antoninus of Florence (archbishop of Florence, 1389–1459) was the first theologian devoting a separate chapter to the various obligations of physicians in his *Repertorium totius Summae* [1]. The first books exclusively dealing with medical ethical judicial (and juridical) questions were *De christiana ac tuta medendi ratione* of Baptista Codronchi (physician at Imola, 1547–1628) [2], *Quaestionum Medico-Legalium Opus absolutissimum* of Paolo Zacchia, (1584–1659, physician general of the Vatican State) [3], and *Ventilabrum medico-theologicum* of the physician and theologian Michael Boudewyns [4]. Among Protestants, medical ethics became a special branch of theological ethics with the Anglican situation ethicist Joseph Fletcher [5] and the more traditional Methodist Paul Ramsey [6].

Nevertheless, Christian tradition has shown an interest in the ethical aspects of medicine from its very first start, which cannot be a matter of surprise, because it always saw a link between disease and healing on the one hand and sin, guilt and redemption on the other. Consequently, disease and healing have been central notions in Christian theology. This is especially expressed in giving Jesus Christ, the Redeemer of all evil, the title 'Christus Medicus', Christ the Physician, who was thus considered the ideal image of the medical doctor.

## Christus Medicus

Though wary of linking disease to personal sin, Christian tradition considers disease and death consequences of original sin. This element of Christian doctrine, especially not explained in very felicitous terms by the later scholastic theologians, can best be elucidated in the way of the Church Fathers (theologians, mostly bishops, in the first six centuries) and the great medieval theologians of the thirteenth century [7]. According to them, original sin consists in a deliberate choice of man to break his initial special relation of friendship and love with God, a condition indicated by means of the image of the Garden of Eden as an earthly paradise, by not recognizing Him as his Creator and Master, and by trying to become equal to Him. The consequence of this was that the first human beings, having lost this original friendship with God and consequently also the special gifts of grace inherent in it, were thrown back on their fragile and vulnerable human nature. Thus, they were exposed to disease and death (Gen 3).

The very core of traditional Christian doctrine is that God, though being one, consists of three Persons: the Father, the Son and the Holy Spirit. The Father sent His Son, truly God, into the world, who being incarnated, that is having become man, died on the cross in order to expiate both original sin and all personal sins. In this way he paved the way for man to be restored to his original dignity, his friendship with God, expressed as becoming a 'child of God', and moreover to participate in the life of the Holy Trinity, ultimately to the full in eternal life after death (cf Rom 5).

The link between disease and sin and faith in Christ as the Redeemer from sin was the basic reason why many Church Fathers gave Him the epithet 'Christus Medicus', though they also promoted this title in order to oppose the cult of Asklepios, the Greek-Roman God of medicine, also venerated as saviour and physician [8]. Moreover, the Gospels report that Christ cured many diseases in a miraculous way during his earthly life as a sign of his being the Son of God, but also as an external sign of the redemption from sin for which he had come in this world. Origen ($\pm$185–254) speaks in his *Contra Celsum* of healing "the whole rational nature and bringing it to familiarity with God the Creator of the universe through the remedy of the Logos (Christ indicated as the incarnated Word of God) [9]." Ambrose (339–397), by way of example, refers to a physician as "having imitated the physician who comes from heaven [10]." He calls Christ a "great physician [11]." Augustine (354–430) most frequently used the title 'physician' in order to describe what Christ did for fallen humanity [12]. In doing exactly the opposite of what the first human beings did through original sin, that is by humiliating himself through his suffering and death, he, the "true physician [13]," became "the complete physician for our wounds [14]."

Because of the obvious analogy between redemption and curing diseases, the title of 'Christus Medicus' was presented in order to explain His mission as a healing ministry especially till the sixteenth century, but also afterwards by both Catholics and Protestants [15]. This image also served as a stimulus for physicians, and for Christians in general, to cure the physical diseases and injuries of the sick with love (philanthropy) and compassion. Philanthropy was already recommended as a characteristic required of the good physician by the Hippocratic writings, Galen and Scribonius Largus (a Roman physician in the first century of the Christian era). Christian Philanthropy is a form of love, the dynamics of Christian ethics in general, which is rooted in the very nature of God (cf 1 John 4,8). This love of God is revealed in Christ's incarnation as unlimited, freely given and sacrificial. Love thus conceived expresses itself not only in curing the patient but also in caring for him, freely treating the poor sick and – perhaps most of all – in attending patients during plague epidemics in a self-effacing way risking one's life [16]. The compassion required is not be confused with superficial pity, but implies sympathizing with and projecting oneself into the position of the patient. Compassion could be nothing else, if it is a form of imitating Christ the Physician who became man and thus shared our existence:

"Since then we have a great high priest who has passed through the heavens, Jesus, the Son of God, let us hold fast our confession. For we have not a high priest who is unable to sympathize with our weaknesses, but one who in every respect has been tempted as we are, yet without sinning ... In the days of his flesh, Jesus offered up prayers and supplications, with loud cries and tears, to him who was able to save him from death, and he was heard for his godly fear. Although he was a Son, he learned obedience through what he suffered; and being made perfect he became the source of eternal salvation to all who obey him " (Heb 4,14–15; 5,7–9) [17].

According to Sigerist, Christianity brought a radical change in the social position of the sick and the organization of health care by society, of which the foundation of hospitals since the last quarter of the fourth century is a clear sign [18].

## The Sanctity of Life

The figure of Christ as physician, as the giver and the healer of life, focuses attention on the meaning and value of human life in itself which is intrinsically related to the dignity of the human person.

His dignity consists in his being a person, having spiritual faculties, reason and will, which account for his ability to make free choices. It is exactly because of his being a person which he owes to his spiritual life principle, the soul, that he reflects something special of his Creator. Thus Genesis, the first book of the Bible says: "Then God said, 'Let us make man in our image, after our likeness ...' So God created man in his own image, in the image of God he created them" (Gen 1,26–27). Because of this special position of man and of the fact that he has as his ultimate end the eternal beatific vision of God, man is an end in himself and not a purely instrumental good. God therefore reserves the right of ownership and the right of disposal of man to himself.

A very important point of Christian doctrine is that human bodily life participates in the dignity of the human person. Though in tradition not all theologians have escaped from a dualistic concept of man, most of them did so following Holy Scripture which regards man as a substantial unity of soul and body. This view is also inherent in the Christian doctrine of the resurrection of soul and body at the end of the world, which means that man will eternally exist as a whole person, not only spiritually but also physically (cf Rom 8,11.23) [19]. One of the first to use the title 'Christus Medicus', Ignatius of Antioch (†107), affirms that redemption concerns both soul and body: "There is only one Physician, both carnal and spiritual, ... Jesus Christ Our Lord [20]."

Using philosophical methods, like that of the Aristotelian-Thomistic tradition by Catholics, supplementary to theological reasoning, Christian theologians were able to respond to what we now term the mind-body problem, the most fundamental problem of Western philosophy. Especially, they managed to avoid the Cartesian dualism, which views man as being composed of two separate components, soul and body. This dualism is – though for the most part unconsciously – the basis of the quite mechanic impact of modern medicine which does not focus on the person as a whole, but on the body as if it were distinct from the person in question. It leaves the care for the spiritual well-being of man to the clergy or – in this secularized century – the psychologist or psychiatrist.

According to the traditional Christian view of man the human body, being an intrinsic part of the human person and thus participating in his dignity, possesses not only instrumental, but also intrinsic value. The stewardship of this world grants man a limited right to dispose of infrahuman nature, but not his own biological nature. God reserves to himself the right to dispose of man's bodily life (cf Gen 9,6). Disposing of something means using it for some self chosen end. This provided Christian tradition with an argument to show that active euthanasia, suicide, infanticide and abortion are incoherent with the whole of its doctrine: these forms of terminating life imply that human life is sacrificed (disposed of) as a means to end suffering. Moreover, its view of the mind-body relation enables Christian tradition to cope with contemporary medical-ethical problems, for instance to regard total brain death as a valid criterion for the death of the human person [21].

Many have reproached the Christian tradition for being contradictory in itself, because it rejects euthanasia and abortion, while permitting killing in just (self)defense and capital punishment, albeit in a very restricted way. If man were the proprietor of his life and had the right to dispose of it, nobody else would ever have the right to take his life. Given the fact, however, that man has only the right to use his life in order to fulfil his duties as human being and as Christian, life can be taken from him if he has lost this right by threatening somebody else's life or the common good (cf Rom 13,1–4). Though it may not be denied that capital punishment and an appeal to just self-defense have frequently been abused, nevertheless the same argument for refuting euthanasia and abortion, namely an accurate analysis of the contents of the right to life, leaves a certain space for killing a criminal whose behaviour is very harmful to the common good and who cannot be punished by life imprisonment.

Manuals of moral theology and medical ethics classified the various forms of terminating human life under the fifth commandment of the decalogue according to the Catholic and Lutheran tradition and the sixth commandment according to Calvinist custom: "Thou shall not kill" (Ex 20,13; Deut 5,17). They also ranked mutilation as falling within this commandment. The principle of totality, which says that a part may be sacrificed in order to save the life of the body as whole, served to explain why surgical operation of the extirpation of organs is no mutilation. The undesired side effects and complications of medical interventions are justified by the principle of double effect: Taking the risk of a negative effect is acceptable if it is not intended either as a means or as an end, in technical terms if it is an 'indirect' effect, and if it is proportioned to the intended therapeutic result.

Another very important issue in the discussion on life terminating acts in Christian medical ethics is the value of suffering. From its very beginning, Christian theology has seen this as a way of identifying oneself with Christ suffering on the cross. Roman Catholic tradition even views it as contributing to the redemption of oneself and others [22]. While the figure of Christ the Physician serves as an identification model for the medical doctor, the Suffering Christ is such a model for the patient. Integrating suffering in one's life by identifying and uniting oneself with Christ has always been a central point of the Christian message. An interesting example is Lidwina of Schiedam (1380–1433), who is venerated as a saint by Dutch Catholics: after having fallen on the ice during skating as a fifteen-year-old girl, she was bedridden for thirty-eight years. Initially she often complained and was a burden to her family. However, by following the advice of the assistant priest of her parish who encouraged her to meditate on the Passion of Christ, she changed gradually but radically into a mature woman, a help and stay for many seeking her advice. This example shows that the Christian faith is not an ideology presenting suffering as a cruel end in itself, but a way of maturation and growth of the human person by being united with Christ for which the integration of suffering in life is seen as a necessary means.

## The Value of Medicine

Thus far, we have only spoken of the sanctity of life as the basis of a negative norm, the prohibition of terminating life to remove suffering. A handicap of medical ethics is often that it mostly deals with the more sensational issues, but quite rarely with the positive every day duties of physicians, nurses and other medical workers. The sanctity of life, implying a duty to preserve and restore it as much as possible, is of course also the basis of their daily work.

Some authors have supposed that early Christianity till the end of the fourth century, did not accept 'secular medicine', that is medicine practiced by the classical Greek-Roman physicians. According to Amundsen

"Many early Christians and Church Fathers, however, insisted that God either inflicts or permits disease and the practition of the secular healing arts thus works against divine purposes. Wide acceptance by the Christians of the medical art as consonant with the sanctified life of faith took centuries. While abortion, suicide and euthanasia became sins, the prolonging of life did not become either a virtue or a duty [23]."

The sources from which this conclusion is derived, are the writings of Tatianus, leader of the Encratites, a very strict ascetic movement during the second century, and Arnobius (North Africa, c. 305). Both had their roots in the gnostic-manichaean dualistic doctrine of Marcion (c. 140) [24], according to which matter was created by the God of the Old Testament, the principle of evil, and the spiritual world by Christ, the God of the New Testament. Hence, they refuted eating meat, drinking wine, marrying and procreating, as belonging to the physical, thus material world. This also included a rejection of secular medicine using material means to cure diseases. Taking refuge in these would mean distrusting God's providence [25]. A refusal of modern medicine has been noted among some Christian groups with regard to the introduction of general anaesthesia during the 1840's. The same applies to the resistance against vaccination of a very re-

stricted number of orthodox Protestants. They read in Mt 9,12 "those who are well have no need of a physician, but those who are sick," and in the definition of Divine Providence according to Sunday 10 of the Catechism of Heidelberg a prohibition of vaccination. Being healthy, man should not take precautionary measures against possible future diseases, because this would imply that he does not recognize God. Man would therefore not be allowed to arm himself with 'non-ordinary' means, such as vaccination, against God's judgements, though he might do so with medicines against diseases, which are regarded as the blows dealt to us by His judgements, according to the text quoted from Matthew. At most, it would be permitted to use 'ordinary' (natural) means, such as sanitary measures, against future diseases [26].

However, all the sources quoted stem from marginal groups in the Christian tradition. Because of his heretic doctrine, Marcion was excommunicated under Pope Pius I as early as 144 [27]. The apostle Paul urges his friend Timothy to drink some wine because of his frequent ailments of the stomach (1 Tim. 5,23). The Book of Jesus Sirach (38,1–15), rated among the books of the Old Testament by the Roman Catholic canon, offers a new and courageous view of the relationship between healing by praying to God and the application of secular medicine. Contrary to Tatianus and Arnobius there are numerous early Christian theologians who appreciated secular medicine very much [28], a.o. Origen [29], Gregory of Nazianze ($\pm$ 330–390) [30], Basil the Great ($\pm$ 330–379) [31] and Gregory of Nyssa ($\pm$ 335–394) [32]. Clemens of Alexandria (140/150-before 216) considers restoring health by means of medicaments as the result of a co-operation between God and man [33]. By their many compilations of antique medicine and their translations of the great ancient medical authors from Greek into Latin and later on from Latin into various vernaculars, the Church Fathers handed over classical medical knowledge to monastic medicine which served as fountains of knowledge for the beginning medieval universities [34].

Moreover, rejecting secular medicine would have been at variance with the essentials of Christian doctrine described above. Redemption does not exclude the physical aspect of man. The best way of formulating the relationship between religious and medical factors in healing diseases is to use the terms in which the Council of Chalcedon (451) expressed the relationship between the divine and the human nature in

Jesus Christ: as these are joined in Him 'unmixed' and 'undivided' [35], one should neither mix secular medicine and healing by prayer, nor separate them totally from one another. The Roman Catholic natural law tradition has always stressed that man, being created in God's image and participating in God's Providence [36], has a serious responsibility, among other things with regard to taking care of life and health. In agreement with the figure of Christ the Physician standing behind the medical doctor, both the Catholic and the Protestant tradition maintained that medicine is to be seen as a continuation of the healing ministry of Christ and a way to fulfilling his command to heal the sick (Mat. 10,8; Luc. 10,9) [37].

However, the conviction that life is an intrinsic good does not imply that it is an absolute good. Prolonging life in hopeless cases reveals in a certain sense the same attitude as that of terminating life in a euthanasia situation, that is the desire to hold the direction of life and death in one's own hands. Thus disposing of them, man refuses to throw himself upon God's tender loving compassion and mercy. The Roman Catholic moralists of the fifteenth century developed the distinction of 'ordinary' and 'extraordinary' means, later formulated as the distinction between proportioned and non-proportioned means as the criterion for evaluating life prolonging treatment: if the ratio between the chance of recovery and the chance of complications and side effects is proportioned, medical or surgical treatment is obligatory; this is not so if this ratio is non-proportioned. If this ratio is disproportionate, treatment should be refused [38].

Another important limit of medical treatment is the borderline between treatment and manipulation. Because of the flagging of the belief in eternal happiness as a life-pervading perspective in Western society due to wide spread secularization, attention is being focussed on health as the most important condition of happiness, even as happiness in itself [39]. This development is rapidly turning health into an absolute good, instead of a relative good. The consequence is that practically every dissatisfaction with physical appearance, not necessarily pathological, is experienced as an illness, an imperfection of the body which should be 'remedied' by modern medicine and surgery. Hence the great interest in body building even by means of hormones or cosmetic surgery. When medical interventions do not have a therapeutic end, but only aim at improving the otherwise healthy body, the body and thus the human person himself is degraded into a

means in order to realize some characteristics deemed to be a perfection and thus happiness. This manipulation, implying a direct disposal of human biological nature, can, however, not be viewed as analogous to the Redemption from evil. Because of this, many patients find it very difficult to accept the message that medicine cannot accomplish anything for them and cannot meet their wishes. By the way, this is also a factor in the growing practice of euthanasia: if health is seen as an absolute good and as happiness in itself, life easily loses its meaning and sense, when health turns out to be 'irreparable'. The only technical means of alleviating suffering would then be the termination of life.

## Conclusion

Though it is often believed that Christianity, superseded and outmoded, cannot offer satisfying or meaningful contributions to contemporary bio-ethical discussions, the opposite is true. Emphasizing that curing concerns the whole person in his spiritual, emotional and physical aspects, a religious tradition such as the Christian can show ways to prevent health care from becoming an overtechnicalised striving for unrealistic physical perspectives alienating man from himself. Instead, it can show a way of becoming a real medical, that is therapeutic cure integrated in the care for the whole person and thus contributing to his true well-being.

## References

1. Antoninus of Florence (1511) Repertorium Summae, compilatus a Joh. Molitore. Basiliae, per Johannem Amorbacchium, Peter et Froben, pars III, titulus VII
2. Baptista Codroncus (1629) De christiana ac tuta medendi ratione. Bononiae, typis Clementis Feronii (first publication in 1591)
3. Paolo Zacchia (1674) Quaestionum Medico-Legalium Opus Absolutissimum. Lugduni, Ex typographia Germani Nanty (first edition in 8 volumes between 1621 and 1650)
4. Boudewyns M (1666) Ventilabrum medico-theologicum. Antwerp, Cornelius Woons
5. Fletcher J (1965) Morals and medicine, 3rd edn. Beacon Press, Boston (first published in 1954)
6. Ramsey P (1970) The patient as person: explorations in medical ethics. Yale University Press, New Haven
7. Grisez G, Shaw R (1991) Fulfillment in Christ. A summary of Christian moral principles. University of Notre Dame Press, Notre Dame/London pp 161–173
8. Rengstorf KH (1953) Die Anfänge der Auseinandersetzung zwischen Christusglaube und Asklepiosfrömmigkeit, Münster: Aschendorff. Rengstorf supposes that Holy Scripture already shows signs of a certain hostility to the Asklepios cult: while

Asklepios was invoked as σωτήρ (saviour) as far back as long before the Christian era, John 4,42 and 1 John 4,14 call Jesus the 'σωτήρ τοῦ κόσμου' (Saviour of the world), thus emphasizing that there is no other saviour besides Him (p 13); another sign would be the battle between Jesus and the Satan called the dragon (δράκων) in the Book Revelation of John, chapter 12: the symbol of Asklepios, the snake, is also termed δράκων; because there was a famous sanctuary of Asklepios in Pergamum in Asia Minor and John is also addressing himself to the church of Pergamum (Rev 2: 12–13: "And to the angel of the church of Pergamum write: '... I know where you dwell, where Satan's throne is'"), Rengstorf thinks that the opposition to the Asklepios cult was at the back of John's mind (pp 25–28)

9. Origen, Contra Celsum 3,54, in: SC 136, p 128; cf 4,15
10. Ambrose, De Cain et Abel 2,3,11, in: CSEL 32$^I$, p 388
11. Ambrose, De Helia e ieiunio 20,75, in: CSEL 32$^{II}$, p 458
12. Arbesmann R (1954) "The concept of 'Christus Medicus' in St. Augustine," Traditio 10, pp 1–28
13. Augustine, De Civitate Dei 4,16, in: CCSL 47, p 112: "Ad quam (quietam) vacat verus medicus dicens: Discite a me, quoniam mitis sum et humilis corde, et invenietis requiem animabus vestris (Mat. 11,29)"
14. Augustine, In Joannis Evangelium 3,3, in: PL 35, col 1397: "... totus medicus vulnerum nostrorum...;" cf. Ibid., 25,16
15. Schipperges H (1965) "Zur Tradition des 'Christus Medicus' im frühen Christentum und in der älteren Heilkunde," Arzt und Christ 11: 16–19
16. With respect to the differences and the points in common between the concept of philanthropy according to the Hippocratic writings and Roman physicians such as Galenus and Scribonius Largus on the one hand and the Christian concept of love on the other, see Amundsen DW, Ferngren GB (1982) "Philanthropy in medicine: some historical perspectives." In: Beneficence and health care, Shelp EE (ed) Reidel Publishing Company Dordrecht/Boston/London II (= Philosophy and Medicine 11), pp 1–31
17. The bible quotations are taken from the Revised Standard Version
18. Sigerist H (1943) Civilization and disease. University of Chicago Press, Chicago, pp 69–70
19. Mondin B (1992) L'uomo secondo il disegno di Dio. Trattato di antropologia teologica. Edizioni Studio Domenicano, Bologna, pp 43–44
20. Ignatius of Antioch (1961) Letter to the Ephesians 7,2, in: The epistles of St.Clement of Rome and St. Ignatius of Antioch, transl. Kleist JA. London, Longmans, Green and Co. (= Ancient Christian Writers 1), p 63 (PG 5,649–652)
21. Eijk WJ (1996) "Het doodsconcept en de doodscriteria." In: Postmortale orgaandonatie. Een medisch-ethische en juridische beschouwing. T. Van Laar (ed) Assen, van Gorcum, pp 13–21
22. John Paul II (1984) "Epistula apostolica Salvifici doloris" (February 11, 1984) Acta Apostolicae Sedis 76: 201–250
23. Amundsen DW (1978) "The physicians obligation to prolong life: a medical duty without classical roots," Hastings Center Report 8, p 27; cf Dawe VG (1955) The attitude of the ancient church toward sickness and healing, doctoral thesis at the Boston School of Theology, pp 153–156
24. Dictionnaire de Théologie Catholique, Vacant A, Mangenot E (red.), (1927) Paris: Letouzy et Ané, vol. IX,II, col 2010–2032
25. Tatianus, Oratio ad Græcos 17–21 (PG 6,841–856); he only conceded the use of medicine as a kind of 'indulgence', ibid., 20 (PG 6,852). Arnobius, Adversus Gentes 1,48 (PL 5,779–781)
26. For analysis of the opposition to poliomyelitis vaccination among Dutch orthodox Protestants see Douma J, Velema J, WH Polio (1979) Afwachten of afweren? Amsterdam, Ton Bolland, (= Ethisch Kommentaar 5)
27. Dictionnaire de Théologie Catholique, op. cit., vol. IX,II, col 2018
28. Frings HJ (1959) Medizin und Artzt bei den griechischen Kirchenvätern bis Chrysostomos, doctoral dissertation at the philosophical faculty of the Rheinische Friedrich-Wilhelm-Universität Bonn, pp 12–17
29. Origen, Explanatio super psalmum 37, homilia 1,1 (PG 12,1369) In: Numoras Homiliae 18,3 (PG 12,715)
30. Gregory of Nazianze, Oratio 28, Theologica 2,26 (PG 36,62)
31. Basil the Great, Homilia 6 in Hexaemeron 9 (PG 29,116)
32. Gregory of Nyssa, De pauperibus amandis, Oratio 1 (PG 46,463)
33. Clemens of Alexandria, Stromateis 6,17 (PG 9,388–390); cf. Origen, Contra Celsum 1,9 (PG 11,673)
34. D'Irsay S (1917) "Patristic medicine," Annals of Medical History, pp 364–378, especially, p 374
35. DH 302
36. Thomas Aquinas, Summa Theologica I–II, 91, 2
37. Ashley BM, O'Rourke KD (1997) Health care ethics: a theological analysis, Washington, Georgetown University Press, 1997 (4th edn) pp 134–135; Verhey, A (1982) "Protestantism." In: Encyclopedia of bioethics, Reich WT (ed) New York/London: Macmillan Library Reference USA/Simon & Schuster and Prentice Hall International, (2nd edn) vol. 4, pp 2117–2126
38. Eijk WJ (1987) De zelfgekozen dood naar aanleiding van een dodelijke en ongeneeslijke ziekte. Brugge, Tabor, pp 156–161, 321–348
39. Viafora C (1998) "Le dimensioni antropologiche della salute. Un approccio filosofico centrato sulla 'crisi del soggetto'," Dolentium Hominum 13, n. 37, pp 16–21

Correspondence: Willem Jacobus Eijk, M.D., Ph.D., Priest, Professor of Moral Theology, Faculty of Theology, Via Nassa 66, CH-6900 Lugano, Switzerland.

Acta Neurochir (1999) [Suppl] 74: 59–60
© Springer-Verlag 1999

# Traditional Ethical Ideas on Life and Organ Transplantation in Japan

**Hajime Handa**

Kyoto University, Takeda General Hospital, Kyoto, Japan

For us doctors, especially neurosurgeons, a day hardly passes without confronting the death of people. However, all people are travelling from birth to death, which is the destination of all our lives. Until a few decades ago, birth and death of people were entirely in God's providence, and medicine was considered to be a discipline to prevent and cure diseases to allow people to enjoy more healthy lives until God calls them. Recently, however, with the remarkable advances of medicine, concepts of birth and death have been diversified and become artificially manipulable. Concerning birth, for example, in vitro fertilization, artificial insemination, surrogate mothers, selection of sex at conception, and planning of the time of birth have become available, and more recently, the production of human clones has become an issue. Concerning death, also, the position to recognize brain death as well as conventional cardiac death as death of an individual has been introduced in association with organ transplantation.

In this lecture, I would like to talk about the state primarily of "brain death and organ transplantation" in Japan.

Brain death is defined as irreversible functional loss of the entire brain in some countries but as irreversible functional loss of the brainstem in others. However, it is universally agreed in that brain death is a state in which cardiac arrest and total death are inevitable with whatever measures to protect other organs. Therefore, although criteria of brain death, and tests to confirm the irreversibility and fatality of the brain damage may vary among countries, they are considered to be essentially uniform.

In Japan, brain death is based on the concept of whole brain death, which is stricter than the criteria in many other contries, and I believe that brain death can be judged unquestionably by this approach.

The Japanese criteria for the judgment of brain death were drafted by a group chaired by Professor Kazuo Takeuchi in 1985 and were presented at the third meeting of the Eurasian Academy of Neurosurgery at Bangkok in 1987.

However, as not a few Japanese people are opposed to regarding brain death as death of a person, discussion has been accumulated for more than 10 years after the announcement of the judgment criteria of brain death. The Organ Transplant Law was finally approved by the Diet on June 17, 1997, legalising resection of organs from brain-dead individuals for transplantaion on October 16, 1997. However, organs can be donated on the condition that the brain-dead individual has a "donor card" stating that the carriers of the cards are willing to donate their organs if they become brain-dead and that their families do not object to donation. Persons aged 14 years or above may have a donor card, and already neary 10 million people are estimated to have donor cards.

Concerning why organ transplantation from brain-dead donors is difficult in Japan in comparison with Western countries, Mr. Taro Nakayama, President of the Diet Committee for Promotion of Organ Transplantation, observed, "Organ transplantation would be difficult in Japan without further deepening of understanding of medicine, law, and emotion." I estimate that Japan is not inferior to other countries in the technique of organ transplantation and that brain death is judged with sufficient accuracy according to reasonable criteria. The problem lies in the characteristic philosophy and view of life of the Japanese based on the lack of complete acceptance of the Western scientific rationalism despite adoption of modern Western medicine.

I understand that the notion, "Once a person dies, the spirit leaves the body, and the body is reduced to a mere object," is generally accepted in the West. As indicated by "Cogito ergo sum" of Descartes, a human being that has lost the ability to think, e.g. a brain-dead person, is regarded as an object, or a cadaver in which the heart, an organ corresponding to a pump, is still moving. Thus, it seems to be rather easy for Western people to accept organ transplants from brain-dead people.

But, in Japan, especially some mothers, when their children become brain-dead, are reluctant to accept the physical state showing warmth and a pulsating heart as dead and unable to agree to donate organs from their brain-dead children.

If I give you another example to show Japanese feeling, even now after 50 years since the end of the 2nd World War, the relatives or the friends of the soldiers killed in war have been visiting Siberia or Southeastern Asian countries battlefields to gather their bones or articles left by them. For the relatives or friends, the bones of soldiers are not only the material but something special in which their spirit still remains. They want to bring them back home and put them into a grave in order to remember the dead.

From my experiences deeply involved in the discussions about brain death and organ transplantation for the past 30 years, I understand that in Japan, "living spontaneously" has been a traditional way of life. Such a thought is observed consistently in Japanese religions, Buddhism, and the spirit of traditional arts.

But, most Japanese people recognize the changes in the concepts of life and death mentioned earlier, and understand the necessity of in vitro fertilization for childless couples and organ transplants from brain-dead donors. On 28th February 1999 – 16 months after the enactment of the Organ Transplant Law – organ transplants (heart, liver, kidneys for 2 persons, and corneas for 2 persons) from a brain-dead donor was performed for the first time. On 12th May 1999, the second organ transplants (heart and kidneys for 2 persons) from a brain-dead donor was carried out. All recipients' conditions have appeared to be good after the transplants, and the organs are functioning properly, doctors said. Kidney, skin, and corneal transplantation from bodies after cardiac arrest and liver transplantation from living donors, who are mostly patients' relatives, are already performed rather commonly. For example, liver transplants from living donors had been carried out in 522 cases (462 children and 60 adults) by the end of 1997 with a 5-year-survival period of about 80%.

In addition to organ transplants, the development of artificial organs, transplantation of tissues or cell cultures from stem cells, and heterogeneous transplantation using transgenic animals have recently been investigated.

In the light of the present state of medicine in Japan, I would like to say in conclusion that application of the latest medical techniques such as organ transplants from brain-dead donors and medical intervention in reproduction should be advanced on the basis of sufficient discussion at a "Bio-ethics Research Conference" in which doctors, jurists, philosophers, religionists, and people in general participated.

Correspondence: Hajime Handa, M.D., Takeda General Hospital, 28-1 Moriminami-cho, Ishida, Fushimi-ku, Kyoto, Japan 601-1434.

Acta Neurochir (1999) [Suppl] 74: 61–63

# Principles and Concepts of Brain Death and Organ Donation: The Jewish Perspective

**Z. H. Rappaport** and **I. T. Rappaport**

Dept. of Neurosurgery, Rabin Medical Center, Tel Aviv University, Israel

## Abstract

The harvesting of organs for transplantation is dependent on a stringent definition of brain death. Different societies have had to struggle with their cultural heritage, adapting it to conform to the advances in medical science and the need of the sick. In this article, the development of the concept of brain death as it applies to organ transplantation in Judaism is outlined. The ability of traditional Jewish values to address themselves to the challenges of modern medicine can serve as a basis for cultural cross-fertilization and comparison in modern societies.

*Keywords:* Brain death; organ donation; Judaism; ethics.

## Introduction

Most of our societies are still deeply influenced by their religious heritage when dealing with ethical issues. Brain death as it applies to organ transplantation is one of the areas most affected by attitudes deriving from social and moral background. In the present article, we examine these aspects in the context of the Jewish religion. A similar process of ethical evolution in other societies has led to the now general acceptance of brain death criteria for the purpose of organ transplantation.

## Background

The sanctity of human life is a cardinal principle of Judaism. One must take every measure to preserve the life of a human being, should it be for a single instant. He who hastens the death of another is seen as a murderer. Therefore, a precise definition of the instant of death is a topic of vital importance in Jewish law (Halakhah). For only the presence of the criteria of death as recognized by the Halakhah relieves a human

being from the obligation to use all available means in order to preserve the life of the patient.

Sources as to the Jewish definition of death are to be found in the Talmud, a vast repository of Jewish law and customs compiled between the 4th and 5th centuries CE. The first case evokes the right to violate the Sabbath in order to uncover a person buried under a pile of rubble [1]. The rescue effort must continue *"however remote the likelihood of rescuing life may be"*, and *"even if found crushed in such a manner that he cannot survive except for a short while"*.

Judaism considers the value of human life to be of infinite value, so that a hundred years and single second are equally precious. However, once it has been determined with certainty that the person has expired, no further violation of the Sabbath is allowed. The question then arises as to how much of the body must be uncovered in order to ascertain that the person has expired. This would obviate the need for desecrating the Sabbath to expose further an obviously dead person. Two opinions are found in the text. The first one states that one must continue to dig until the nose is uncovered. If there is no sign of respiration, the person is declared dead. The second opinion deals with the situation in which the body is uncovered from the feet up. If one arrives at the chest and no heartbeat is found, death can be declared. This, however, remains a minority opinion. The authors felt that a faint heartbeat might be mistaken for an absent one, whereas determination of the absence of respiration was a far more robust sign of death. The centrality of respiratory cessation in determining death is based on the biblical sentence: *"... all in whose nostrils is the breath of the spirit of life [2]"*. In fact the Hebrew word for soul, *neshama*, is closely related to the word for respiration, *neshima*.

The second Talmudic issue of relevance permits the desecration of the Sabbath in order to perform a Caesarean section so as to save the life of a foetus whose mother died in childbirth [3]. The 16th century rabbinical authority, Rabbi Moses Isserles questioned this Talmudic directive. He denied that there was sufficient medical competence in his time to ascertain the exact moment of the death of the mother. The possibility therefore arises that the operative intervention might hasten the demise of the mother and be equivalent to murder [4]. This statement, however, admits exceptions. Thus Rabbi Yaakov Reisner states unequivocally: "*The physician who had the presence of mind to incise the abdomen of a pregnant mother who was decapitated on a Sabbath, so as to save the fetus, should have no pangs of conscience, since in this instance the mother's prior death is established beyond doubt*". In this case the very short continuation of the heartbeat is not considered as residual life but as "*the twitching of an amputated lizards tail or the death throws of a decapitated man*", meaning "*manifestations of cellular life that continued after the death of the entire organism had occurred* [5]". With these exceptions, the consensus was to rely upon respiratory cessation in determining the moment of death. Stopping of heartbeat occurred within minutes of respiratory arrest. Absence of heartbeat was therefore seen as a sign that respiration had irreversibly disappeared.

## Present Attitudes

These criteria were unproblematic until the 1960s. However, with the introduction of artificial respiration, cardiac activity could be maintained for a prolonged period in the absence of spontaneous respiration.

Rabbinical authorities had to deal with novel questions: When is it acceptable to turn off a respirator, without being responsible for murder? Is heart transplantation acceptable? On the one hand, one cannot say that the artificially ventilated patient has stopped breathing. One could view the removal of his heart as tantamount to murder. Furthermore, in its initial days heart transplantation was a very hazardous procedure. For the recipients there was a significant risk that the procedure might shorten rather than prolong life. It was suggested that the transplant procedure is actually a double murder, that of the donor and that of the re-

cipient [6]. On the other hand, if the potential donor is truly dead, there is a mandatory religious obligation to use all means to save or prolong the life of the recipient.

There was initially a considerable resistance among rabbinical authorities to except the then novel criteria of brain death, especially in their use for determining the potential for organ donation. However, as the success of heart and liver transplantation increased, the question was re-examined from a Halakhik point of view. Brain death similarly to prolonged cessation of the heartbeat was interpreted as a sign that the absence of respiration is permanent.

In 1987, the Chief Rabbinate of Israel accepted the performance of heart transplantation in Israel, based upon the declaration of brain death of the donor. The establishment of criteria was handed over to scientific experts with participation of a member of the Rabbinate. The criteria at that time included the following points:

1. Knowledge of the cause of illness.
2. Complete cessation of spontaneous ventilation.
3. Clinical demonstration of the destruction of the brain-stem.
4. Objective support of the clinical determination by brain-stem auditory evoked potentials.
5. Demonstration that absent respiration and brain-stem activity persist for at least 12 hours under full therapy.

## Brain Death in Children

There is essentially no difference in the Jewish religious attitude as to the criteria for ascertaining death in children versus adults. If medical authorities would propose more stringent criteria for declaring brain death in the child, this would serve as the basis of the religious determination.

As regards to foeticide, Judaism has a somewhat different approach when compared to classic Catholicism. The Scriptural basis of this approach relates to the case of an inadvertent injury to the foetus during an altercation between two men:

"*And if men strive together, and hurt a woman with child, so that her fruit depart, and yet no harm to follow, he shall be surely fined, according as the woman's husband lays upon him; and he shall pay as the judges determine. But if any harm follow, then shalt thou give life for life . . . [7]*".

The Jewish interpretation of this passage is that as long as "no harm follows" for the woman, there is no capital offence involved in the killing of the foetus. The Christian interpretation is based upon a mistranslation into Greek in the Septuagint, where "*no harm to follow*" is rendered "*[her child be born] imperfectly formed*". The distinction between an unformed and a formed foetus and branding the latter as murder was accepted by Tertullian and by later Church fathers. The distinction was subsequently adopted in canon law as well as in Justinian Law [8]. Since 1588, the Catholic Church has viewed the killing of a foetus as murder from the moment of conception [9].

Jewish Law maintains the full title to life to start only at birth. In the Talmud embryotomy is sanctioned if the mother's life is endangered:

"*If a woman is in hard travail [and her life cannot otherwise be saved,] one cuts up the child within her womb and extracts it member by member, because her life comes before that of [the child]. But if the greater part [or the head] was delivered, one may not touch it, for one may not set aside one person's life for the sake of another [10].*"

The later rabbinical responsa deal with the question of dismemberment of the embryo even during the final stages of parturition. Even if the mother's life is endangered by an impacted breech delivery, embryotomy is sanctioned if the majority of the foetus has been delivered. This ruling applies to the situation when both the mother and the foetus would die without this manoeuvre. During the first 30 days of life, in the Jewish view, an infant is in a status of having to prove that it is viable. Thus, parents must not halakhically mourn the death of an infant within this time frame. There is therefore an inequality between the mother's life, which is established, and that of the infant who has yet to prove its viability. This difference is usually of no significance, and does not allow for killing of the infant to save the mother's life, except when both are doomed to die without the intervention.

If this type of argument is applicable to the well-publicised case of hydranencephalic infants serving as organ donors, is not yet certain. Certainly Jewish religious authorities in the past have proved themselves able to deal with the demands which modern medicine continuously imposes on society's ethical traditions.

To quote an old Yiddish proverb:

"*Ever since dying has come into fashion, life hasn't been safe.*"

## Acknowledgement

This paper was presented in part in a symposium on religious attitudes towards brain death organized by Dr. J. Haase (Aalborg, Denmark) during the 14th Meeting of the European Society of Pediatric Neurosurgery, Lyon, France, September 1994.

## References

1. Babylonian Talmud, Yomah 85a
2. Genesis, 7: 22
3. Babylonian Talmud, Arakhin 7a
4. Orech Chaim, Question 8
5. Gilon Hadassa (1969) Letter from Jerusalem, defining death anew. Science News 95: 50
6. Shut, Agrat Moshe, part Yoreh
7. Exodus 21: 12
8. Westermarck (1939) Christianity and Morals, 243
9. Bonnar (1948) The Catholic Doctor, 78
10. Mishna Tohorot II, Oholot 7: 6

Correspondence: Z. H. Rappaport, M.D., 49100 Petah Tiqva, Israel.

Acta Neurochir (1999) [Suppl] 74: 65–68
© Springer-Verlag 1999

# Brain Death in Practice – A Retrospective View

## E.-O. Backlund

Department of Clinical Neurosciences, Neurosurgery Section, University Hospital, Linköping, Sweden

In my country, Sweden, the concept of 'brain death' was not accepted formally by the law until 1988, after a long and partly heated debate, even an agitated dispute within the medical community itself. Now, after more than 10 years, the debate still has a tendency to flourish occasionally, and, interstingly, opinions thus expressed by the lay public have gradually influenced both the legislative process and the practice, for example the introduction of a voluntary Donor Card system.

This presentation is a kind of very personal and thus subjective eyewitness' report from the first decade of 'brain death' in Sweden, a country officiously protestant, however secular to a degree today typical for 'western countries'.

The basic ethical question, i.e. *under what principal conditions* any organ might be 'disposable' for retrieval, was hardly raised by the spokesmen for 'brain death'. The Swedish Government, obviously afraid of fuelling a debate biased by the 'supply-and-demand-of-transplants' aspects, appointed a committee which was given the specific task of investigating the possible need of a concept of death *founded on principle, completely removed from* the potential implications for transplantation surgery. This basic frame of reference seemed to be an implicit attempt to disinform the Swedish people, and moreover it made the committee's work factitious. At least, it forced the investigators into a non-biological argument. This was what remained when the search for tenable arguments supporting the 'brain death' concept *in a biological paradigm* proved to be elusive. The introduction of such an artificial concept of death would not have become necessary, if the basic ethical questions had been approached and answered first.

For the lawmakers, the following daring deduction became necessary: If a 'dead-to-be' person could be formally declared dead before his organs were destroyed by the lack of oxygen (induced by a heart arrest traditionally constituting death), this situation would allow retrieval of organs, *given that organ retrieval from dead individuals is acceptable in principle*, from an ethical point of view. This deduction is hardly surprising. In the post-mortem room, doctors have long become accustomed not to worry about possible ethical objections when organs are removed from corpses, for scientific or educational purposes. The rationale now was that organs from 'brain dead' patients might be taken on the same grounds.

During the Swedish debate, some leading neurosurgeons, as well as many ICU and OR nurses, were among those who strongly objected to the 'brain death' concept as a criterion of death. This was probably a key factor in producing the polarization of standpoints that followed. Medical personnel who have direct responsibility for a potential organ 'donor' are most often the people who naturally express the most pronounced objections. On the other hand, those most actively advocating the new concept of death were often found, apart from those being far away from any patient, for example philosophers and experts on ethics, among neurophysiologists, anaesthetists and, of course, transplant surgeons.

In retrospect, the 'brain death' concept, applied to *practice*, has clearly revealed its poor foundation in biology, in patient management and in common sense. Further, and most important, *it is not a prerequisite for organ retrieval*. It is indeed surprising, that so many countries accepted a law-founded 'brain death' concept obviously without first addressing the basic ethical questions. They seem to have accepted, almost axiomatically, dubious principles of proprietary rights allowing society to harvest human organs from an individual *as soon as he/she is declared dead.*

In a country like Sweden, dying and death have gradually become 'institutionalized'. Fewer people than are commonly supposed have actually *seen* a dead peson, i.e. a corpse. When it comes to 'brain dead' patients, only the closest relatives of such an individual have the opportunity to become acquainted with this fortunately unusual situation. Moreover *few physicians* will have experienced a 'brain death' situation, a surprising fact to the non-medical community. Thus, only an extremely small number of people will have had the opportunity to see a 'brain dead' person. Indeed, this holds true also for those who most vividly take part in public discussion on the topic, ethicists, politicians and press people. Legislators may have theoretical knowledge of the biological background of 'brain death', but no practical experience. The public debate which has ensued strongly indicates that the inexperienced will have great difficulty in recognising what this condition means in practice.

Dying has, during the history of man, fundamentally and always been a common event, a completely natural part of human life. This is clearly a positive and very important factor. It is crucial that any one person is competent to judge whether a fellow-man is alive or not. When situations of dying and death have to be met, there is a definite human value in communicating what is happening in simple and adequate layman's terminology. The ability to understand and recognise that a person has 'lost his life' should not be an issue for experts. But this does not mean that the state of death should not be *confirmed* by an expert. Under all circumstances, one must by all means avoid turning the state of 'being dead' into a *diagnosis*, which can only be recognised by qualified experts, after examination. The death of a human being is, and must remain, an event familiar to the common people.

*Medical practice in general* has no need for a new concept of death. This contributes to the fact that legislative committees fail to raise any arguments other than philosophical ones. For example the essential conclusion made by the Swedish committee was the following: As each individual human brain *constitutes a human individual*, a patient without a vital brain must be considered a 'non-individual', i.e. a dead person, irrespective of the condition of the rest of his body, including organs other than the brain. From a purely biological, 'materialistic' point of view, this is absurd. The body of a 'brain dead' person is *in the literal sense*

harbouring *vital* organs, even vigorous enough for a 'second life' in the body of another person!

The reason for introducing a term like 'brain *dead*' was obviously to avoid possible but *selfevident* objections from the laity, namely that the body of a 'brain dead' person is not *truly* dead. People realize, for example, that all the measures usually performed with corpses, transport to the mortuary and autopsy, etc., are completely out of question with a 'brain dead' persons. The 'brain dead' donor-to-be is rather an intensive care patient, subject for ambitious treatments. Professor Lars Leksell, my principal mentor and close friend for many years, himself an active opponent to 'brain death' as a criterion of death, put it this way: "A person is not dead until he or she can be sent to the mortuary". This ingenious statement is a sovereign definition of death, based as it is upon practical circumstances, mature clinical experience, and upon common sense.

The concept of 'brain death put into practice may give rise to the most absurd situations, of which some examples are given here. With one exception (the case of a pregnant woman), they are from my perssonal experience:

## Dead and Living Patients may be Together in a Hospital Ward

Of two neighbouring patients in an ICU, one may be declared formally dead and the other alive. A dying, but *formally living* fellow-patient of a 'brain dead' person, next to him in the room, may be looked upon as a meaningless case, with all treatment judged as pointless and thus under withdrawal, whereas qualified and even expensive therapy is spent upon his *formally dead* neighbour, to make his organg as fit as possible for the grafting procedure. It is not difficult to find such a situation offensive. Hospitals have the duty to provide a mortuary for patients who die, but it is repugnant to the fundamental idea of a hospital to treat dead individuals in a ward, together with ordinary patients.

## A Physician can Choose his Patient's Hour of Death

As soon as the investigations show global and irreversible damage to the patient's brain, it is up to his doctor to eventually decide (within certain limits) *when* the patient should 'die formally'. If this happens around midnight (or even more crucial at the turn of a year), this might cause unwanted judicial and practical consequences as the date (or year!) of death can be decided on by the physician.

## Uncertainty may Prevail Among Nurses as to Whether a Patient is Dead or not

Communication between teams changing duties under stressed conditions, often characterizing the work in an ICU, may be less satisfactory, and the result from an examination verifying 'brain death' may accidentally be 'lost' in the nurses' reporting. "What did the doctor say, is Mr X dead or not?" should be an unthinkable question from a nurse, nowadays however completely possible.

## A Newborn's Hour (Date) of Birth may be set Later than his/her Mother's Moment of Death

The case of a 'brain dead' pregnant woman with a full-term unborn baby has become a 'classic'. Any problems in such a case might be judicial only, but so far, at least in my country, this issue does not seem to have been approached by lawyers.

## From a Strictly Judicial Point of View, it Would Today be Possible to Use 'Brain Dead' Patients for Research and Education in the same Manner as Corpses

For the purpose of research or education, physicians habitually do not hesitate to 'profit' from the fact that patients die. The positive importance of this for the progress of medicine is obvious. Post-mortem measures such as surgical training in connection with routine autopsy have been widely accepted as ethically tolerable. To suggest something similar in a 'brain dead' individual should by everybody be expressed as a flagrant violation of the 'brain dead' person's integrity. This contradictory parallell illustrates clearly that a 'brain dead' individual is *not a dead person in the real sense*.

## The Collaboration Between Physicians Responsible for a 'Brain Dead' Patient may be Disturbed by Disagreements

A doctor may refrain, for psychological or other reasons related to the case in question, from being too active regarding organ retrieval. He or she may be more inclined to just switch off the ventilator, to 'give up', and let the patient 'die in peace'. The reluctant doctor might then be accused by colleagues of a lack of humanity, of begrudging potential organ recipients a better or longer life. This is a painful experience for this doctor when his/her essential arguments for being reluctant are related to psychological subtleties noted in the family of the dying patient, not fully recognised by the other doctors involved.

It is notable that transplanted organs as a rule are called 'donor organs' although a fundamental uncertainty prevails concerning the factual conditions in the individual retrieval situation. In public polls, around 20% may be found opposed to the idea of donating organs after death and a large group remains undecided. In Sweden, after public information and using the present 'Donor Card' system, only about 50% of the population has explicitly agreed to give their organs after death. Our judicial regulations originate from the assumption that *presumed consent* is a self-evident popular attitude, which obviously is far from the real situation. Thus in an individual case, an organ transplanted today may have been 'taken' from a 'supplier' rather than 'given' by a 'donor', should an agreement on the individual's Donor Card be missing.

To conclude, and importantly, it is completely possible to meet the demands of transplantation surgery without the 'brain death' criteria. Ethical demands are met if organs for transplantation always and consistently are given *voluntarily* and the donor can do without the organ(s) in question. Based upon this principle, it should be possible to formulate a kind of universal declaration for *any* donor, conscious and healthy, *or* 'brain dead' and thus dying (Fig. 1). Such a Magna Charta might be formulated as: "*I am still alive*, and *I give my organ(s) voluntarily*, because *I can do without it (them)*". Such a statement corresponds completely with a 'Yes' on any 'Donor Card'. A voluntary agreement from the 'brain dead' donor, given any time during his/her previous conscious life, would allow organ retrieval to be performed *without violating ethics*, and, most importantly, *without any preceding declaration of death*. Philosophical objections regarding the latter have been raised. It has been argued that the removal of a still beating heart, from a patient who

1. I am still alive *and*
2. I give my organ(s) voluntarily *because*
3. I can do without it (them)

Fig. 1. The Magna Charta of Organ Transplantation. A Universal Declaration by Any Donor

is formally alive, i.e. the 'brain dead' individual, in theory must be considered a murder. As the medical community now is well acquainted with and accustomed to withdrawal of therapeutic measures in completely hopeless cases, also in cases other than 'brain dead' patients, this argument is without relevance. There is no appreciable *ethical* difference between switching off a ventilator removing a beating heart, both procedures representing nothing but the ultimate surrender in a case far beyond any chance of survival.

As a matter of course, I have myself been instrumental in promoting a number of organ retrievals. But *I cannot recall a single case*, where it has been actual, useful or even necessary to use the 'brain death' concept as a fulcrum for the family's decision to allow donation. The decision has always been considered reasonable and well-founded *because of the literally hopeless prognosis, and not due to any artificial assumption that the 'donor' is dead*. To a closely related kin, the general impression of the 'brain dead' relative in his/her bed never leads to the conception of a corpse.

It is remarkable that transplant surgeons do not seem to appreciate the potential future risks for their speciality, as long as the occurrence of 'brain dead' patients is an important prerequisite for the availability of organs. The near future may well show a sophisticated method for a fast, easy and reliable diagnosis of 'brain death' already at the emergency entrance, with the injuried person still on the ambulance stretcher. There are good reasons to believe that such an unfortunate fellow-man will never be admitted into any hospital as a 'dead patient' for treatment, exclusively as a donor-to-be. This aspect means a formidable challenge to transplantation surgery already today.

Moreover it is a challenge for the international neurosurgical community to help the public, politicians and legislators to fully appreciate problems and questions of a kind raised in this review. Practical experiences from our clinical departments and common sense deserve to be regarded as the most important and even crucial factors in any retrospective evaluation of the 'brain death' concept as applied in practice. The perspective is now long enough to make a reassessment of this issue not only reasonable, but highly desirable.

Correspondence: E.-O. Backlund, Department of Clinical Neurosciences, Neurosurgery Section, University Hospital, Linköping, Sweden

Acta Neurochir (1999) [Suppl] 74: 69–70
© Springer-Verlag 1999

# Criteria for Selection of 'Death with Dignity' – From Clinical Cases of Malignant Brain Tumours

**M. Nagai**

Department of Neurosurgery, Dokkyo University School of Medicine, Japan

## Introduction

Recent rapid progress in medicine has brought into focus a number of bio-ethical issues regarding life and death of human beings. Among the most common and most controversial problems in medical ethics are those involving the termination of life support. Neurosurgeons also frequently confront difficult situations in which serious decision-making is required.

In this paper, the bio-ethical concept of 'death with dignity' is discussed in the context of three patients with malignant brain tumours.

## Case Report

### Case 1

A 75-year-old man, Professor Emeritus of Engineering. In August 1988 he complained of a headache and left hemiparesis. On admission, malignant lymphoma of the right deep frontal lobe was diagnosed by brain imaging. His prognosis was explained to him. He showed us his advance directives which included refusal of surgical treatment including blood transfusion. For this reason, only radiation and steroid therapy were started, which markedly reduced the tumour volume in the first month. Then the patient refused the continuation of radiation therapy, and enjoyed his hobby, painting, and the pleasure of life with his family. In November, steroid therapy was also stopped because of its adverse effect of a gastric ulcer. In December, the patient refused even drip infusion of liquids, and the disease progressed to the point where his consciousness level was depressed; this was followed by 4 months of terminal care in a lethargic state.

In April 1989, the patient died with serenity, without using a respirator, according to his family's request.

### Case 2

A 36-year-old woman. Her initial sign was a defect of the visual field. In December 1994, a stereotactic biopsy was done at a university hospital and glioblastoma of the thalamus was diagnosed. Subsequent radio-chemotherapy had little effect. In May 1995, the patient came to our university clinic in a bed-ridden state. Her husband refused active or aggressive treatment for her and desired home care rather than admission to the hospital. He had previous experience with terminal care of malignancy, since his former wife had died of stomach cancer. Immunotherapy was initiated using a monoclonal antibody for glioma. The patient was treated at home, with occasional visits to the outpatient clinic over six months. She died calmly in the hospital three days after admission for fever and respiratory distress.

### Case 3

A 13-year-old girl. Gait disturbance was the initial sign, which appeared in June, 1983. Six months later, an extensive removal of a cerebellar tumour was performed at a university hospital. The histopathological diagnosis was malignant ependymoma. Postoperative radio-chemotherapy was administered. Subsequently, the patient attended school for ten years in a state of remission. In June, 1993, ten years after the onset of the disease, the patient complained of a headache. Brain imaging revealed recurrence of the tumour, which enlarged rapidly and invaded the brain stem.

In September 1993, she was admitted to our hospital in a bed-ridden state. Marked cerebellar ataxia and paralysis of the lower cranial nerves were noticed but she remained conscious. Her parents were fully informed about her illness and her chances for survival. Based on this information, they refused any treatment other than terminal care. About two months later, she died peacefully in a state of general weakness.

## Discussion

The three cases presented here raise numerous bioethical issues. Refusal of active or aggressive treatment was a common theme in all three cases. In case 1, the patient himself prepared his advance directives, which made it simpler to withhold aggressive treatment. In cases 2 and 3, the patient's spouse or the parents also refused any active treatment. A decision not to leave home was made in case 2 according to the family's wishes. In case 3, the parental right to make a decision regarding their child was a serious point to be discussed. These medico-ethical problems focused attention on the criteria for selection of 'death with dignity'. According to the definition of the Japanese Association for Death with Dignity, Death with Dignity is equivalent to passive euthanasia and is an act which brings one closer to the natural course of death. The authors use the term in this meaning. The problem is how and when we should select death with dignity. Emanuel [1] stated that the following factors should be taken into account when deciding whether to withhold life support or withdraw active treatment; the chances for successful treatment; the projected quality of life; and the predicted survival of the patient.

'Death be not proud' is a famous book written by John Gunther during the course of his son Jonny's disease, and published in 1949. Jonny, a 17 year-old boy who suffered from glioblastoma, had been treated by every conceivable means in the period just after the second world war. At the end of the book, Gunther noted that "Jonny did not die like a vegetable. He died like a man, with perfect dignity". Today, 50 years after this story, how far have the treatments for glioblastoma advanced? In spite of the development of therapeutic approaches for this tumour, how long has the survival of the patient been prolonged? Based on these considerations, the authors would like to propose the following criteria for selection of 'Death with Dignity': 1) patient has received therapy for controlling all depressive symptoms; 2) prolongation of life is hopeless from the view point of quality of life for the patient; 3) complete informed consent is obtained from the patient, or from surrogates when the patient is incompetent or is of younger age group; 4) a team approach to decision making has been organized. These four conditions are essential to the concept of death with dignity.

## Conclusion

Although several advanced therapeutic regimen are being developed for treating malignant brain tumours, the prognosis is hopeless for some patients. They should be allowed to die with dignity after all other options have been considered.

## References

1. Emanuel EJ (1994) Objections to the best interest standard. Ends of Human Life. Harvard Univ. Press, Cambridge, London, p 74

Correspondence: Masakatsu Nagai M.D., Department of Neurosurgery, Tochigi Red Cross Blood Center, 4-6-33, Imamiya, Utsunomiya, 321-0192 Tochigi, Japan.

Acta Neurochir (1999) [Suppl] 74: 71–74
© Springer-Verlag 1999

# Death With Dignity – On the Withdrawal of Life-Sustaining Measures

**E.-O. Backlund**

Department of Clincal Neurosciences, Neurosurgery Section, University Hospital, Linköping, Sweden

The methods for diagnosis and treatment have today reached a degree of refinement and efficacy which tends to make them too powerful tools in our hands, when dealing with critically ill patients. In top-equipped hospitals, it is not quite uncommon to witness processes of dying more extended than what should be natural in a biological, psychological as well as ethical perspective. To use our formidable diagnostic and therapeutic capacity in a reasonable fashion is indeed a challenge, not least to the less experienced doctor or nurse. With a scent of black humour, someone in my country recently made this very pertinent remark: "The progress in medical research has increased the average age of man, by lengthening the process of his dying".

At least in our society, modern man seems to have lost his ability to look upon death and dying as completely natural parts of human life. Contributing to this is the fact that the eventual phases of many people's lives occur in hospitals and nursing homes. Moreover the icon of the Perfect, Healthy and Attractive Human Being is cherished, particularly among young people. When Man is looked at from the perspective of the healthy, active and vigorous individual, any old, probably dying and thus 'useless' care-taker might be regarded as a disturbing factor in his/her mind, causing panic and anxiety, apart from any fundamental subconscious death agony already present . This is indeed a challenge to our educational system, among others. At least in my country, the lower grades of the elementary school may have missed the chance to include discussions on existential issues, and on the fundamental conditions of being a human person, in their non-physical aspect.

Medical doctors are hardly exceptions from people in common. Their minds may also harbour anxiety and fear when death and dying are met. To me, *two patterns of attitude* are easy to recognize. In an subconscious attempt to "defend his/her mind", one physician may be staying in the corridor, in front of the door of a room housing a terminal patient, when the daily prescriptions should be dealt with, during the routine round in the ward. This doctor tries to escape from his/her agony by a kind of neglect, in a mind where even vague thoughts about passive mercy-killing might be discernible. Neither is a kind of inverse pattern uncommon. In this case, the physician tries to cope with his/her agony by 'over-treating' the dying patient, in an unconscious attempt to hinder the process of dying, not seldom by recommending spectacular therapeutic measures, literally useless if not even violating the patient's integrity.

Also in Sweden, we have a branch of the Exit movement, the international network for the promotion of assisted suicide. From one of its founders, by the way a close friend of mine, I learned that the reason for establishing this branch in Sweden was that so many hopelessly ill and/or dying patients were not 'allowed' to die with dignity in hospitals and homes for the elderly. Lots of useless 'therapeutic' measures were employed, in the individual case sometimes violating the personal integrity and the patient's right to 'decease in a normal manner'. This might be an expression of a wide spread but subconscious frustration, among the personnel of these institutions, towards the fact that the final phase of a man's life necessarily must include suffering, decay, separation and, eventually, death.

Among these patients, there are some who suffer more then others, for example those who have pain which is unbearable and resistant to 'pain-killers'. This should speak in favour of an 'over-treatment'. But obviously this therapy is not adequate. It would be unfair to deny that a few of these patients desperately ask for physician-assisted suicide. But we have learned from colleagues exclusively dealing with terminally ill patients in hospices and nursing homes, that an attentive attitude, an ambitious individual refinement of the pain medication, the use of psychological support, and probably the offering of a confession, most often makes any potential discussion on physician-assisted suicide less relevant.

It is inevitable to include some words about the term euthanasia in this context. In the ordinary person's mind, this word most often is associated with concepts like 'killing'. Surprisingly, also many physicians and nurses prove to be less familiar with the *literal* meaning of the Greek term. An adequate translation into English might be "to die under optimal conditions" or "to die well". Two attributes have been coined for use together with this concept, 'active' and 'passive' euthanasia, respectively. It is of the utmost importance, at least for anyone in medical practice, to be familiar with the *virtual* definition of these two concepts, and it is *crucial* to distinguish between them. This is the more important as the Exit movement seems to intentionally aim at obscuring such distinction, thus facilitating the arguing for mercy-killing.

In 'active' euthanasia the evident purpose is to bring about 'the condition of being dead'. The basic principle is 'relief from suffering by killing'. The aim is to *interrupt the patient's process of life* when the latter is judged as unbearable. Notably, this judgement might be significantly influenced by others than the patient him/herself. Moreover in a recent study of a group of patients 'qualified' for discussion of physician-assisted suicide, more patients than was assumed proved to have a psychiatric depression which could be cured, making the discussion on euthanasia less real (Lancet 347: 1805–1810, 1996).

In our country, most people seriously engaged in medical care find arguing for 'active' euthanasia offensive, and not rooted in what is defined as 'care'. Moreover it is very difficult to conceive and even accept a situation, when a legislation of 'active' euthanasia gives any patient a princial right to physician-assisted suicide upon request, and moreover forces physicians to accept the duty to effectuate this, on a matter of official business.

So-called 'passive' euthanasia refers to something radically different. The basic principle is 'to refrain from prolonging a natural process of dying'. The term relates to a kind of 'capitulation' to the inevitable, to the fact that, in an individual patient, it is not only reasonable but ethically correct to surrender, to stop 'treatment' in vain, and to welcome the imminent and natural death. My personal preference is to completely avoid using the word 'euthanasia' in such cases, being a term with a too dramatic a taint. There is nothing sensational in a clinical situation when a physician takes practical consequences of a virtually hopeless situation, into account by refraining from prolonging the patient's dying.

When discussing 'passive' euthanasia with my students, I have found the following metaphor useful. I learned from a friend of mine, an air pilot, that the completion of any air flight is divided in three procedural phases, 'approach', 'descent' and 'landing' (Fig. 1). '*Approach*' essentially needs no explanation, during the approach the minds of the crew is increasingly occupied by the fact that the goal comes nearer. The navigational standards for keeping the plane steady following a route are tapered down to one single aim, namely to have its direction finely adjusted towards the site of arrival. Important is, however, that the pre-planned approach *may be exchanged* for anoather approach, even to an alternative airport, should weather conditions or other unexpected factors give reason for this. It is not too late for those who supervise and govern the air traffic to give an order for another landing site.

Neither deserves the term '*descent*' a thorough explanation. The route has now to be changed in the vertical dimension, and the exact position of the air field will now be plotted onto the landing radar screen. Surprising factors may however again appear, and the fact that the descent has been initiated, does not *absolutely* mean that the pilot has an unconditional permission to proceed to the landing strip. Every frequent flyer is familiar with the fairly common practice of a number of turns over a crowded or foggy airport, time-consuming, useless for the passenger, but inevitable for acceptable security.

'*Landing*', however, is characterized by being the *one single alternative*. The speed and the direction of the aircraft must now, without any change, satisfy rigorous safety measures, and the only tolerable termination of the journey is that the wheels of the aircraft are set onto the ground as accurate, safe and confortable as ever possible. And importantly: *No* phase of a flight is as demanding as the landing. Although sophisticated instruments give an excellent support, the attention of

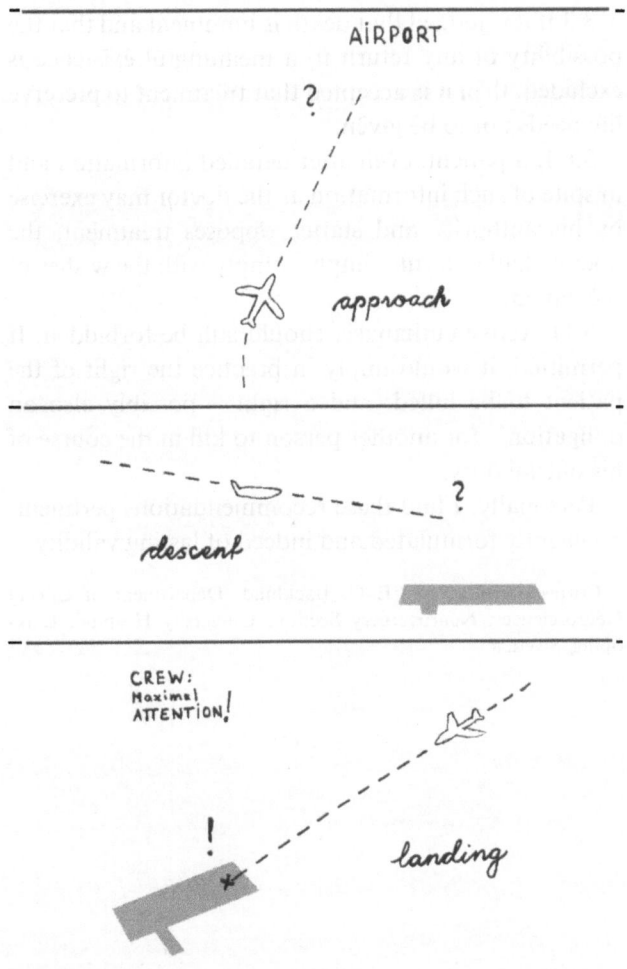

**Fig. 1.**

the crew has now to be at its absolute maximum. If ever, during a long and, for the captain maybe demanding flight, he or she must now be alert. His/her responsibility for a happy end of the journey has no margin for bargaining.

Now take the example of a patient with a glioblastoma. In the moment when you have the painful but delicate task to inform the patient about his/her serious disease, *approach* has begun. In spite of the supposed very poor prognosis, the *true* eventual fate of the patient however remains obscured, both by deceptive expectations but also by possible, factual and/or potential alternatives. In terms analogous with the flight situation, and being the patient's 'pilot', you must check that the goal becomes appreciable for all involved and that the therapeutic 'direction' is correct. But you will not be able to give any quite firm predictions regarding the next course in detail. Unex-

pected things may happen and, at least, the time for the 'arrival' cannot be settled with accuracy.

To continue with the analogy. The *descent* phase begins when you have to tell the patient about a recurrent tumour. A gross removal was performed without problems, the postop oncological treatment went well, but nevertheless: the most recent CT scan *was* disappointing. Still, the rest of the flight is literally unknown, it might be necessary to circle around the airport at a lower level for a time. The arrival *may* be delayed – somewhat. But you have to reassure the patient that you have the continued course safely under control, in spite of an inherent unpredictability, regarding the details.

For the experienced neurosurgeon, there are no problems about recognising the symptoms and signs indicating the beginning of the *'landing'* phase, in a patient with a glioblastoma. Here is, above all, where we have to learn from the flight analogy. It is now that the doctor and his staff have to mobilize all their interest in, and direct all their attention to the patient. I think that few of us can fully stand a retrospective self-examination on this specific point.

This relates to the key issue when 'passive' euthanasia is considered. There is, in the framework of 'maximal attention', a natural and obvious room for surrendering. There is nothing dramatic in this. Notably, *the essence of* 'passive' euthanasia is present in *all* our work, probably without our thinking of it. The daily work of any physician is to *repeatedly take the fate of his/her patient in his/her hands*, by innumerable decisions, trivial as well as fatal: "Antibiotics or not? Pain-killers or not? Referral to another expert or not? Operation or not? Radiotherapy or not?". The most fateful decisions are of course those which have directly to do with the patient's life and death, for example the answer to the question: "Ventilator or not?".

To 'give up' pointless medical 'treatment' during the very last hours of the 'landing' phase is an important constituent in the maximum attention the patient deserves. It has nothing to do with 'killing' or so-called 'active' euthanasia, it is euthanasia in its literal sense, 'to die under optimal conditions'.

For me personally, it is striking how little we learn about these things during even a long professional life. When it comes to what I like to call 'surrendering', it is impossible to achieve full 'competence', applicable in *any* patient's case. You will never be able to free yourself from the absolutely unique and often subtle psychological relation which you have to the individual patient. Neither can you escape influence from the common combination of confidence and despair, expressed by the family. But with sensible fingertips and with maturity, it is nevertheless often possible to choose a route of 'surrendering', hallmarked by realism rather than rationalism.

Already 20 years ago, a report from a governmental expert board in Sweden gave excellent guidelines regarding the problems discussed here (SOU 1979:59, State Department of Sweden). To regret, these recommendations seem to have been forgotten or are disregarded by the Government today, as a similar board has been commissioned recently. I would like to give credit to the first board of 1979 by quoting some crucial items from their report:

3.1 The basic rule is that the patient has the right to decide for himself whether or not he wishes medical care. In principle, he must decide for himself what treatment he is prepared to undergo.

3.3 If it is judged that death is imminent and that the possibility of any return to a meaningful existence is excluded, then it is accepted that treatment to preserve life needs not to be given.

3.6 If a patient, even after detailed information and in spite of such information as the doctor may exercise by his authority and status, opposes treatment, the doctor shall as a rule simply comply with the wishes of the patient.

3.11 Active euthanasia should still be forbidden. If permitted, it would imply in practice the right of the patient to be killed, and a right – possibly also an obligation – for another person to kill in the course of his official duty.

Personally, I find these recommendations pertinent, excellently formulated and indeed of lasting validity:

Correspondence: Dr. E.-O. Backlund, Department of Clincal Neurosciences, Neurosurgery Section, University Hospital, Linköping, Sweden.

Acta Neurochir (1999) [Suppl] 74: 75–81
© Springer-Verlag 1999

# Euthanasia in the Netherlands: Transparency and Accountability

**R. Dillmann**

Royal Dutch Medical Association, Utrecht, The Netherlands

## Introduction

The practice and regulation of euthanasia in the Netherlands is often used in debates concerning legalization of euthanasia (or physician assisted suicide). The situation in the Netherlands has both been used as a deterrent, and as a support for legal changes elsewhere [1, 2]. The scope of this contribution is not to influence these debates. The goal is to give an overview of the current situation in the Netherlands, without suggesting that the way euthanasia is regulated in the Netherlands is an export product. This, however, does not imply that euthanasia and physician assisted suicide are not an international issue. They are, because patients and physicians in many countries are confronted with it. Euthanasia and physician assisted suicide pose a clear challenge to the medical profession, since it is not to be expected that the issue will disappear by itself.

There are three reasons why the practice and regulation of euthanasia and physician assisted suicide in the Netherlands are not to be seen as an export product. The first is that the practice of euthanasia (physician assisted suicide included) cannot be separated from the quality of the system of health care. It is particularly important that decisions to perform euthanasia are free from constraint and coercion, and do not come about because of deficiencies in health care. Since the quality and accessibility of systems of health care differ greatly among countries, this implies a clear warning against generalizing the practice and regulation such as it has come about in the Netherlands. The specific nature of our system of health care has been described elsewhere quite extensively [3]. Some characteristics are worth mentioning: an extensive system of general practitioners, a large number of nursing homes, nursing home medicine as a distinct specialty, a high level of pain treatment, and – increasing – attention for palliative care. In addition to this everybody is insured for the costs of protracted illness, and thereby financial incentives do not play a role in the treatment of and care for patients who are dying.

The second reason is the role of the medical profession. Since the 1970s the relationship between physician and patient became more egalitarian, and less paternalistic. This is a development which is not unique for the Netherlands, but it has taken a specific form in our country. Patients are critical about the role of their physician, but also respect his or her knowledge and skills. Patients rights have been laid down in a bill of patient rights, and patients tend to get involved more and more in the decision making process. On the other hand the medical profession in our country has made it an important point in its policies to be clear and transparent about its practices. These two elements (i.e. an egalitarian relationship between physician and patient, and the wish of the medical profession to be transparent, thereby realising a relationship of trust) are of overwhelming importance in view of the practice and regulation of euthanasia.

The third reason – less tangible – is the importance of particular cultural values in the Netherlands. In general Dutch culture has an egalitarian character, with tolerance for different viewpoints and lifestyles. This is connected with a strong sense of solidarity – also in the context of health care insurance. This brings about a tendency to government regulation, resulting in a fine maze of rules, regulations and laws. These are, especially regarding medical ethical problems, based on broadly shared views, respecting the freedom of those who judge differently [45].

Although euthanasia has to be seen within the

context of each country and its cultural and moral community, the fact remains that euthanasia is an international issue. In many countries patients ask for euthanasia and assisted suicide, and physicians do respond to those requests. In the literature, reports can be found concerning Australia, the UK, the USA, and Denmark (see Table 1). The precise findings are difficult to compare owing to the different methods used, and the wordings of the questions, but in general a substantial part of the medical profession has faced a request for euthanasia, and a significant proportion has performed euthanasia (or has provided the pharmacological means for assisted suicide). In the State of Oregon (USA) for instance 21% of the responding physicians had received a request for euthanasia in the past year, and 7% had prescribed a drug in compliance with this request [6]. In a national survey in the USA it was found that 18% of physicians had received a request for assisted suicide, 11% for a lethal injection, and 8% said they had complied with these requests [7]. In the United Kingdom Ward and Tate found that 60% of GP's and hospital consultants had received a request for euthanasia or assistance in suicide and 14% had performed euthanasia [8]. These data show that euthanasia and physician assisted suicide belong to the reality of medicine in many countries.

**Euthanasia: Definitions and Frequencies**

In the Netherlands euthanasia is defined as ending the patients life by the administration of drugs, at the patients explicit request. Although euthanasia and physician assisted suicide differ in practice, in the Netherlands both acts are considered to be morally equal. In both cases we deal with acts on behalf of the physician, resulting in the death of the patient. It can be argued whether or not there is a difference between the two: is acting different from enabling? If one enables the patient, then the last cause of death, is the patient's act. This is different from euthanasia. In both cases, however, death is intended, and realizing this intention by acting or by enabling is difficult to distinguish. Nevertheless, there are two relevant differences. The first is that in the case of enabling there might possibly be less reason for doubt regarding the true wish of the patient. This is of course of a relative nature, especially when the true nature of the wish of the patient has been established in a correct way. The second is that the moral burden for the physician might be less, since the final act is the patient's. This draws also on the assumption that the moral burden might be influenced by whom the act is performed. The responsibility in both cases is however equal, and the only difference might be that the risk of coercion and abuse is less great in the case of physician assisted suicide. In general it might be more sensible to put trust in proper ways of regulation, review and control, in order to restrain coercion, than in these somewhat theoretical distinctions. To give a better impression of these technical data, two case descriptions can be found on next page.

Euthanasia and physician assisted suicide must be differentiated from ending of life without an explicit request, i.e. the administration of drugs with the explicit intention to end the patient's life without an explicit request by the patient. In these cases the patient has discussed his wishes previously, but at the time he or she lost consciousness, and was not able to reconfirm his wishes. Another possibility is that there was no previous discussion or wish known, but that the situation had become such that it was decided to intervene actively. In general this is done by the administration of opioids in dosages that surpass therapeutic levels.

The last type of medical decision related to the end of life is increasing pain and symptom medication by the administration of opioids with a probable life shortening effect.

Table 1. *Euthanasia and Assisted Suicide Internationally*

| | Country | Received request for euthanasia or assistance with suicide | Willingness to take active steps if it were legal to do so | Complied at least once |
|---|---|---|---|---|
| Lee et al. 1996 | USA | 21% (in the last year) | 46% | 7% |
| Meier et al. 1998 | USA | 29% | 36% | 8% |
| Emanuel et al. 1996 | USA | 57.2% (oncologists) | — | 13.6% |
| Ward & Tate 1993 | UK | 60% | 46% | 14% |
| Kuhse & Singer 1987 | Australia | 48% | 40% | 29% |
| Baume & O'Malley 1993 | Australia | 47% | — | 28% |
| Folker et al. 1996 | Denmark | 56% | — | 7% |

*Case 1*

A 56 years old female patient stays at home after extensive treatment for breast cancer. The tumour has spread to the bone marrow, her spine and possibly to the brain. Pain control is optimal, symptomatic radiation of the spine took place. Nevertheless the patient suffers from pain and other symptoms. After repeated requests the GP consults an independent physician, who visits the patient and checks upon the medical care. The GP also consults the oncologist to check whether or not there are other possibilities for alleviating her symptoms. Three days later the GP performs euthanasia in the presence of her husband, her children and some friends. The case is reported to the legal authorities.

*Case 2*

An 80 year old male patient suffers from end stage cardiac failure, after 3 myocardial infarctions. He is bedridden, and cannot walk. He suffers from permanent dyspnea. A recent stay in a specialised clinic proved unsuccessful in realising a higher cardiac output. After repeated requests and a second opinion from a cardiologist, his GP decides to assist in suicide.

## The Ethics of Euthanasia

The ethics of euthanasia and physician assisted suicide is characterized by two conflicting principles. The first is respect for biological life, the second is respect for biographical life. Often it is argued that medical ethics prohibit physicians from performing euthanasia or assisting patients to die, on the basis of the Hippocratic oath, and the sanctity of life. The sanctity of life argument has, however, a clear vitalistic flavour. The mere presence of biological life – the force of life per se – in a human being is interpreted as a clear moral objection to euthanasia. It is on the other hand quite clear that in modern interpretations of life human personhood as a unique manifestation of biological life, has a strong moral relevance. Someone's life history, his biography, encoded in his body and his brain, resulting in his wishes and preferences are unique manifestations of human life. If someone has a well considered wish for euthanasia or assisted suicide, then this might overrule the principle of respect for biological life. In essence the more complex from of life (personhood) can overrule the lesser complex form of life (the presence of the force of life as such).

This is the moral background of the practice of euthanasia in the Netherlands. There are situations in which a living person urgently requests to have his or life ended when further living has become unbearable, meaningless and disgracing, when prolonged suffering overcomes the positive meaning of life. To follow such a wish is an act which expresses respect for human life and human dignity.

## Challenges for the Medical Profession

Euthanasia poses a challenge for substantial parts of the medical profession. There are at least two reasons for this challenge: 1) the fact that patients have these requests, 2) the fact physicians comply with these requests. In general it is accepted that euthanasia is not part of regular medicine: it is not a patients right, but a doctors favour. In granting this favour fundamental principles are involved. The transgression of the basic medical rule to respect life requires evidence of high quality decision making. This evidence can only come about by being transparent about these decisions, and to be accountable for them. Hence the quality of the decision making process and the quality of the care provided are of fundamental moral importance. This requires two things: transparency and accountability.

## Transparency

Transparency has in the Netherlands come about by two nation wide investigations into medical decisions related to the end of life, respectively in 1990 and in 1995 [9, 10]. Some of the data from these studies are summarised in this section and in tables (2–5). As far as these data are concerned two aspects are important: the facts, and the trends (i.e. 'the slippery slope'). The data will be discussed briefly before we interpret them in view of the slippery slope.

The number of cases of euthanasia in the Netherlands was estimated to be 2.3% of cases of death in 1995 (1.9% in 1990, see Table 2). Physician assisted suicide concerned 0.4% of cases of death (0.3% in 1990). In 0.7% active ending of life without an explicit request took place (0.8% in 1990). Administering of opioids in large doses, such that it was probable or foreseeable that life was shortened happened in 18.5% of cases of death in 1995, and 17.5% in 1990.

Regarding cases of active ending of life without an explicit request it must be noted that in 52% of these cases euthanasia had been discussed previously, but that the patient was not able to give an explicit concurrent request. The drugs used were opioids in 81% of cases, indicating that these cases were near alleviating pain and other symptoms. In 91% the time by which life was shortened was less than a week. Cases of active ending of life of neonates belong also to this category. In general these acts take place after a decision to forgo treatment has been taken, resp. 8% and 57% of all cases of death among children under 1 year [11].

Table 2. *Euthanasia, Assisted Suicide and Other Practices at the End of Life in the Netherlands*

|  | 1995 | % | 1990 | % |
|---|---|---|---|---|
| *Number of deaths* | *135.500* | *100* | *128.800* | *100* |
| No medical decision | 78.600 | 58 | 79.800 | 62 |
| (Unexpected death) | (42.000) | (31) | (38.600) | (30) |
| *Active ending of life* | *4.500* | *3.4* | *3.700* | *2.9* |
| Euthanasia | 3.200 | 2.4 | 2.300 | 1.8 |
| Physician assisted suicide | 400[1] | 0.3 | 400 | 0.3 |
| Without explicit request | 900[2] | 0.7 | 1.000 | 0.8 |
| *Opioids in large dosages* | *25.100* | *18.5* | *22.500* | *17.5* |
| With the intention to accelerate death | 4.100 | 3.0 | 4.500 | 3.5 |
| Accepting the possibility of hastening death | 21.000 | 15.5 | 18.000 | 14.0 |
| *Decisions to forgo treatment* | *27.100* | *20.0* | *22.500* | *17.5* |
| With the intention to accelerate death | 17.600 | 13.0 | 11.000 | 8.5 |
| Accepting the possibility of hastening death | 9.500 | 7.0 | 11.500 | 9.0 |

[1] Including 2 to 5 cases of assisted suicide performed by a psychiatrist.
[2] Including 90 to 95 cases in which the life of a newborn was ended, in 80 of them after treatment was stopped.

Table 3. *Reasons for a request for Euthanasia or Assisted Suicide*

|  | Main reason (%) | Mentioned (%, more than one answer possible) |
|---|---|---|
| Unbearable suffering | 35 | 70 |
| Loss of dignity | 22 | 50 |
| Prevention of further suffering | 5 | 40 |
| Life is pointless | 10 | 38 |
| Pain | 13 | 27 |

These data can be compared with data regarding Australia. Kuhse *et al.* found that of all Australian deaths, 1.8% concerned euthanasia and assisted suicide (2.7% in the Netherlands). Ending of patient's life without a concurrent explicit request amounted to 3.5% (0.7% in the Netherlands) of all deaths [12]. Alleviation of pain with opioids in doses such that a life shortening effect was probable came about in 30.9%.

In Table 3 the reasons for a request for euthanasia or assistance in suicide are listed. In general pain is rarely the main reason for euthanasia, and in many cases more than one reason is relevant. In Table 4 The reasons for the rejection of a request can be found. All in all about 30% of requests end in euthanasia or assisted suicide. There are several reasons for this but two issues are pivotal: 1) the condition of the patient and the presence of alternatives, and 2) the well-con-

Table 4. *Reasons for the Rejection of a Request for Euthanasia or Physician Assisted Suicide*

| | |
|---|---|
| Suffering not unbearable | 35% |
| Treatment alternatives available | 32% |
| Depression | 31% |
| Objections physician | 20% |
| Request not well-considered | 19% |
| Patient lacking insight in disease | 16% |
| Non-voluntary request | 10% |

sideredness of the request, such as in cases of clinical depression.

Patients receiving euthanasia have cancer in 80% of cases (compared with 27% of overall mortality). 70% of cases of euthanasia and 98% of cases of assisted suicide are performed by general practitioners, implying that patients stay at home. This comes about as a rule after extensive clinical treatment proved ineffective.

## A Slippery Slope?

Usually two versions of the slippery slope argument are distinguished: a conceptual and an empirical version [13]. The conceptual version holds that accepting practice A logically implies, either direct or stepwise that practice B, which is morally unacceptable, has to be accepted too. Therefore practice A has to be rejected. The empirical version is that a particular practice, once accepted, will lead to the acceptance of other practices, by gradually changing peoples opinions, leading to an important and undesirable change in society. In practice however we are dealing with the empirical version of the argument, since logic is in general not enough to go from practice A to B.

Furthermore two points must be distinguished: accepting the fact that physicians assist actively in dying, and legalising this practice. Many hold the view that euthanasia is part of medical practice, although against the law. It is not this fact which they fear, but the fact that legalising euthanasia would set off changes which cannot be controlled. Therefore we have two slopes: morally accepting euthanasia, and accepting legalisation of euthanasia or assisted suicide.

In the Netherlands several findings suggest that – so far – things are not out of hand:

– From 1990 to 1995 there were 37% more requests for euthanasia at a later time, and 9% more explicit requests at a particular time. The total number of

deaths increased by 5%. The incidence of euthanasia increased from 1.9 to 2.3%. This is in part explained by the increase of the cancer death rate. In general a clear, but relatively small increase in cases of euthanasia can be observed.
- A decrease in active ending of life without an explicit request from 0.8 to 0.7%.
- No extension to other categories of patients: the number of psychiatric cases is quite small (2 to 5 patients in 1995 and they also had a serious somatic disease), euthanasia concerning demented patients is equally rare, active ending the life of comatose patients does not take place.
- The opinions of the Dutch public have so far not shifted into a more permissive attitude [14].
- The practice of physicians indicates a steady increase in the adherence to the procedural requirements (consultation, case report, notification).

Comparing the Dutch data with those from Australia, then we see that, the overall frequency of active assistance in dying by physicians is 3.4% in the Netherlands, and 5.3% in Australia. Moreover the proportion of active ending of life without an explicit request is 0.7% in the Netherlands and 3.5% in Australia. Although many reasons might exist for these differences, they at least do not indicate that the approach in the Netherlands (accepting euthanasia both morally and legally) leads to a slippery slope. If that were the case then the Dutch figures should be higher than the Australian ones.

## Accountability

Euthanasia is a sensitive issue, involving the transgression of basic moral rules. In view of this it should be taken for granted that physicians are accountable for the decision making process and the resulting actions regarding euthanasia or physician assisted suicide. This implies that a proper system of review, consultation and control should be in operation to guide the practice of euthanasia. The elements of the system as it exists in the Netherlands are: 1) the material requirements 2) consultation, 3) notification, 4) review and 5) control on the basis of a legal framework.

## Material Requirements

The material requirements concerning euthanasia are to be found in a body of jurisprudence, built over the years via numerous court cases, with a few exceptions brought about to gain legal clarification. The requirements are:

- The patient considers her suffering unbearable and hopeless. The physician has to support the viewpoint of the patient on the basis of her clinical expertise.
- There are no realistic treatment alternatives present. This implies that a request for euthanasia fails if the patient refuses a reasonable medical treatment.
- The wish of the patient is well-considered and persistent. If the patient appears clinically depressed then consultation by a psychiatrist is necessary (and treatment of the depression).
- The request must be voluntary (preferably supported by an advance directive).

## Consultation

Consultation by another independent and competent physician is necessary. This physician should interview and investigate the patient, and review the case, including the quality of care given. The consultant should review the patient record, and form an opinion about any (palliative) alternatives left. The consultant, in order to retain his independence, should not be a relative of the attending physician, should not be his employee, or his partner in a practice. A special protocol has been developed for performing a consultation, and for making a report. The report of the consultant is part of the case-report and should be handed over to the legal authorities.

From Jan 1st 1999 a national network of specially trained consultants under the auspices of the Royal Dutch Medical Association will get into action. This is the follow-up of a pilot project in the Amsterdam Region (Support and Consultation with Euthanasia in Amsterdam – SCEA) [15, 16].

## Notification and Review

After euthanasia or assisted suicide took place the legal authorities should be notified. In practice the physician reports to the coroner. This is a legal requirement on the basis of the Burial Act. The coroner informs the public prosecutor, who in turn gives permission for the burial of the body. In table 5 an overview can be found of the number of cases reported since 1981. Clearly, the number of cases reported in-

Table 5. *Cases Reported to the Legal Authorities 1981–1997*

| Year | Reported cases | Cases discussed in assembly | Inquests + dismissal | Prosecutions | Court decisions |
|---|---|---|---|---|---|
| 1981–1985 | 71 | NA | 1 | 8 | 1 acquittal |
| 1986 | 84 | NA | 1 | 2 | 2 acquittals, 1 suspended sentence |
| 1987 | 126 | NA | 1 | 3 | 1 acquittal plus fine, 1 discharge |
| 1988 | 184 | NA | 1 | 2 | 2 suspended sentences (1 with a fine) |
| 1989 | 338 | NA | 2 | 1 | 1 acquittal with a fine |
| 1990 | 486 | NA | 2 | 1 | |
| 1991 | 866 | 14 | 0 | 1 | 1 discharge |
| 1992 | 1201 | 17 | 2 | 2 | |
| 1993 | 1304 | 26 | 11 | 4 | 2 acquittals |
| 1994 | 1487 | 27 | 6 | 5 | 1 acquittal, 2 guilty without punishment |
| 1995 | 1466 | 36 | 3 | 1 | 1 acquittal, 3 suspended sentences, 1 guilty without punishment |
| 1996 | 1832 | | | | |
| 1997 | 1907 | | | | |

creased until a level of about 60%. Since November lst of 1998 the case is then reviewed by one of 5 regional multidisciplinary review boards, composed of a jurist, an ethicist, and a physician. If the case is reviewed favourably, then the commission informs the physician within 6 weeks. The prosecutor will come into action if the review board considers the case to be irregular.

## Legal Framework

Currently euthanasia and physician assisted suicide are forbidden by the law, with sentences of 12 respectively 3 years of imprisonment (Dutch Penal Code section 293 and 294). The Burial Act requires physicians to report (formally illegal) cases of euthanasia and assisted suicide to the legal authorities. In addition to this the government has installed regional review boards for reported cases. All in all this is a paradoxical situation, both from the legal and from the medical perspective.

In the elections of 1998 the current coalition partners in the Dutch government agreed upon a change in the Penal Code, implying that euthanasia performed according to the material and procedural guidelines would not be prohibited. If the physician does not comply with the guidelines, however, then he or she will confront criminal charges. This proposal of law is currently being studied. It is expected that this proposal will come into force within the next two years. Only then the paradox mentioned above will disappear, and a sound basis for review will be realized. Retaining euthanasia and physician assisted suicide in the Penal Code will inevitably compromise the notification rate.

## Conclusions

Euthanasia and assisted suicide in the Netherlands should not be used as a deterrent or a support for legal changes elsewhere. Not as a deterrent, because the situation in the Netherlands is not on a down-hill slippery slope [17]. Not as a support, since the situation in each country is different, and each moral community has to come to terms with this issue on its own. Nevertheless we should conclude that euthanasia is an international issue, since patients in many countries ask for euthanasia, and many physicians comply with these requests. It is foreseeable that these questions will not go away by themselves, and therefore the medical profession is being confronted with a real challenge. The challenge to take care of dying persons as well as we can, including all possibilities palliative care has to offer, and the challenge to respond to requests for euthanasia, which are a reality of contemporary medicine.

In the literature a shift can be observed from debating the ethics of euthanasia, towards the ethics of a system which reviews, controls and regulates euthanasia. I would suggest that the most important ethical question at the time is not whether or not euthanasia in morally acceptable, but how to realize a morally sound practice of euthanasia. To realise transparency and accountability, a system of quality assurance is necessary. The moral issues involved require, however, that such a quality system has a legal backbone. Such a system should leave ample opportunity for realizing feedback between the reviewers and reviewed, and more importantly, it should stimulate the formation of medical ethical rules about the proper practice of euthanasia and/or assisted suicide. In such a system professional and independent review of the case before euthanasia takes place is crucial.

## References

1. Hendin H (1997) Seduced by death: doctors, patients and the dutch cure. Norton, New York
2. Angell M (1996) Euthanasia in the Netherlands – good news or bad? NEJM 335: 1676–1678
3. Schrijvers *et al* (1997) Health care in the Netherlands, Ambo, Baarn
4. Grifftihs J, Bood A, Weyers H (1998) Euthanasia & Law in the Netherlands. University Press, Amsterdam, pp 9–13
5. Pijnenborg L (1995) End-of-life decisions in Dutch medical practice. Thesis, Erasmus University Rotterdam, pp 119–132
6. Lee MA, Nelson HD, Tilden VP *et al* (1996) Legalizing assisted suicide – views of physicians in Oregon. NEJM 334: 310–315
7. Meier DE, Emmons CA, Wallenstein S *et al* (1998) A national survey of physician assisted suicide and euthanasia in the United States. NEJM 338: 1193–201
8. Ward BJ, Tate PA (1994) Attitudes among NHS doctors to requests for euthanasia. BMJ 308: 1332–1334
9. van der Maas PJ, van Delden JJM, Pijnenborg L (1991) Euthanasia and other medical decisions concerning the end of life. Lancet 338: 669–674
10. van der Maas PJ, van der Wal G, haverkate I *et al* (1996) Euthanasia, physician assisted suicide, and other medical practices involving the end of life in the Netherlands, 1990–1995. NEJM 335: 1699–1705
11. van der Heide A, van der Maas PJ, van der Wal G *et al* (1997) Medical end-of-life decisions made for neonates and infants in the Netherlands. The Lancet 350: 251–255
12. Kuhse H, Singer P, Baume P *et al* (1997) End-of-life decisions in Australian medical practice. MJA 166: 191–196
13. van der Burg W (1991) The slippery slope argument. Ethics 102: 42–65
14. van Holsteyn J, Trappenburg M (1997) Het laatste oordeel. Meningen over nieuwe vormen van euthanasie. Ambo, Baarn
15. Philipsen B, van der Wal G (1998) Steun en consultatie bij euthanasie in Amsterdam. EMGO, Amsterdam
16. Onwuteaka-Philipsen BD, Kriegsman DMW, van der Wal G *et al* (1999) GP's opinions on consultation of another physician in case of euthanasia (submitted for publication)
17. Angell M (1996) Euthanasia in the Netherlands – good news or bad? Editorial. NEJM 335: 1676–1678

Correspondence: Dr. Rob Dillmann, Secretary Royal Dutch Med. Ass., Lomanlaan 103, 526 D Ultrecht, The Netherlands.

Acta Neurochir (1999) [Suppl] 74: 83–87

# New Technologies and Methods in Neurosurgery – Ethical Dilemmas

## T. Trojanowski

Department of Neurosurgery and Paediatric Neurosurgery, University Medical School, Lublin, Poland

## Introduction

Progress in neurosurgery, like in any other medical discipline depends nowadays on very elaborate, complex and expensive research. This is driven by the natural curiosity of man, his endeavour for improvement and by competition. There is no doubt that those forces lie at the basis of the great achievements the medical profession is proud of and which, most importantly, benefit the patients.

In the course of funding new ideas, testing them and applying clinically there are many traps and temptations which may lead to conscious or unintended violations of ethical rules. I happens that new discoveries in biology and medicine, the significance of which is often difficult to determine, go beyond human imagination and confront societies and professionals unprepared philosophically, mentally and legally. It is disputed whether law should defend primarily the rights of an individual, of the society or an abstract idea of progress for the benefit of mankind. Contemporary societies value rather individual well-being and rights then the scientific progress.

A good example of challenges in the ethical evaluation of progress in medicine is provided by successful cloning of animals which created concerns related to cloning of man. This new situation surpasses the existing legislation and new paragraphs need to be added to the existing ethical codes and conventions. Similarly transplantation to the human brain was raising a lot of controversies in the past. Loew pointed out that resolution of new ethical issues is not quite so complex if certain well established rules are followed. Among the most important he indicated need for sufficient basic research preceding clinical trials, good design of the

trial, multidisciplinary co-operation in well selected centres, informed consent, absolutely no premature release of information to public media [6].

In neurosurgery the great majority of novel methods of treatment require very expensive instruments, drugs and equipment. It is enough to mention new sophisticated imaging diagnostics, some radiation or chemotherapy protocols, surgical instruments linked with navigation or robotic devices, implants. They are obviously not available to everyone, patients and neurosurgeons, and this is one of the important sources of ethical dispute and numerous lawsuits. It is questionable if mere possession of the newest technology and modern equipment warrants professional promotion. Regretfully there are examples when access to new devices is used for unjustified, commercially motivated claims. Neuronavigation could serve as an example of a new technology that introduces progress into surgery of the brain and spine but as a result of aggressive promotion and intellectual fascination becomes overestimated as an indispensable neurosurgical tool. In fact the great majority of operations will probably remain to be executed without electronically guided neuronavigation without compromising safety or outcome. One of the prominent neurosurgeons irritated by overestimation of the role of presently available neuronaviagtion systems stated: brain is not an ocean, neurosurgeons do not need navigation but a thorough knowledge of anatomy.

A side effect of the publicity given to the new attractive methods are inquires from patients about technical aids used during neurosurgical treatment proposed to them and sometimes refusal of consent for treatment if no lasers, ultrasound, computers or similar instruments are to be used. Contemporary societies give credence to the power of human mind and technology, and are easily misled by unrealistic claims on novelties in medicine particularly if they are supported with scientific sounding theories. A neurosurgeon's obligation is to counteract such claims.

## Research and Progress

Research is the basic source of progress. It is now characterized by high cost and institutional and legal control. There are also problems in carrying out research the involving human person.

The Code of Ethics of the Philippine College of Surgeons states in art. IV sec 3 that the surgeon undertaking experimental and research surgery must be guided by approved protocol for such study. A worldwide inquiry made by Poza in relation to various aspects of neurosurgical ethical codes disclosed very many neurosurgeons expressed an opinion that the control of new drugs and devices should be made by the ministry of health, universities and various committees. It is a matter for institutions and not for neurosurgeons.

### Consent for Experimental Treatment

Difficulties in communication due to dysphasia, disturbed comprehension or consciousness occurring in many neurosurgical patients affect the process of obtaining informed consent for surgery [10]. It is even more complex when a proposal is made to a patient to enter a randomised study with a chance that he/she will be receiving placebo. There is an unresolved controversy as to how unconscious patients can be entered into trials, particularly when the therapeutic time window is narrow and there is no time to refer to the court or legal representatives. Moreover there is legislation which requires, unlike in the case of consent for treatment, that consent of an incompetent patient to participate in a trial be given only by the court, and not by his/her legal representative.

Submission is particularly difficult in trials of new treatments which should be administered as soon as possible in patients who unexpectedly become unconscious as a result of brain insult or injury. Referring to courts or finding legal representatives involves a delay which negates the potential benefits of the drug or treatment to be tried. If a properly tested substance with preliminarily established positive activity and safety could not be given in the acute stage of the disease to unconscious patients for whom they were designed, no progress in the treatment of those conditions could be achieved. There are some agreements of the ethical authorities in Europe, that such experiments are possible if there is minimal risk involved and a clear potential benefit for the patients exists. There are however countries where experiments involving incompetent patients and particularly children are extremely difficult or even impossible to conduct.

### Organisation and Financing of Research

New methods of treatment must be properly, scientifically evaluated taking into consideration both the benefits and complications. An economic approach to health services is clearly in conflict with experiments and developing new treatments. In the times when medical services are organised to be most efficient also from the economic point of view, the majority of departments have no interest in carrying out clinical research. It usually requires more staff, additional examinations, documentation and longer hospital stay which increases the cost of treatment. There are similarly restraining effects on treatment protocols aimed at the most efficient use of resources. They limit opportunities for modifications or development of new treatments as a result of the risks of litigation when the protocol is not followed strictly [9]. The legal requirement of practice according to a responsible body of opinion, expressed in the Bolam rule, should not however arrest the constant search for improvements and innovations in medicine [3]. Most research is contemporarily driven and financed by the industry. The motivation and ethics of commercial corporations differs from that of the medical profession. They also have different goals.

Scientists and companies work under a high pressure of time and competition which may result in various medico-legal problems bound up with the introduction of new procedures into clinical practice. This usually resulg from lack of adequate basic research before entering clinical trials, too short a follow up, premature reporting in the public media or even in reputable journals of inadequately confirmed results. Too early or over-enthusiastic publications sometimes lead to demands from the public or health authorities for the use of procedures without adequate critical assessment of the results. The psychological situation thus created is often very troublesome. One must admit that it is difficult to deny a desperately ill patient with no hope, use of a new procedure of yet unproven value. Mass media are very eager to publish information on new achievements in medicine. Every year the media disclose unjustified claims being made and solutions promised to the patients. The harm such premature or totally wrong publicity does to patients and to the medical profession is reflected by inclusion of paragraphs on this issue into many ethical codes and guide lines. It is a general rule that the results of research on new technologies and procedures should be first published in peer reviewed scientific journals and that pressures from the public and media should not be accepted [4]. Premature release of unproven results of new treatments to the media is regarded as unethical by the Code of Ethics of the Philippine College of Surgeons, which requires in art. II sec 4 that "Achievements in medical science shall be published only in legitimate medical journals". Appropriate chapters on this issue can be found in the Code of Ethics of the American Association of Neurological Surgeons, Guide for Good Practice prepared by the WFNS and EANS and many others.

Surprisingly it is not a common practice of the scientific journals to require from the authors any confirmation that the studies involving human subjects were done in agreement with the code of ethics. Of the 102 English-language biomedical research journals listed in the 1995 Abridged Index Medicus, 47% required institutional review board approval of studies involving human subjects as a prerequisite for publication, 24% did not present or refer the author to any information related to human research ethics, 15% referred authors to the Uniform Requirements for Manuscripts Submitted to Biomedical Journals, 3% to the Declaration of Helsinki, and 10% indicated that informed consent should be obtained [1].

In order to avoid mistakes and unjustified claims based on poor research it is quite common to require that testing of the new procedures is done only in the appropriately equipped and staffed centres under close supervision of national or international professional societies, research and ethical committees. This evolution changes traditional freedom of every doctor to do research in the field of clinical medicine. Pioneers are forced to justify new clinical methods and be subjected to consultation and peer review of the aims, objectives and training requirements. If this is followed then the Bolam rules help to protect an individual in case of litigation [3].

## Maintenance of Knowledge and Competence

New procedures are not minor modifications of the existing methods, but are so different from the current practice that they require special training.

The Code of Ethics of the American Association of Neurological Surgeons (http://www.aans.org) in paragraph IID requires that the neurological surgeon shall be actively involved in continuing medical education to keep up to date on new medical technology and information in neuroscience. Similarly the Code of Ethics of the Royal Australasian College of Surgeons in paragraph 15 obliges surgeons to be informed of new knowledge concerning the art and science of medicine.

Chapters on the necessity of achieving and maintaining surgical competence and of keeping up to date are present in literally all medical codes of ethics.

Neurosurgeons should submit their work for regular review by clinical audit and change the surgical practice as a result of such review. There is also a duty to react to inadequate practice of neurosurgical colleagues.

Responsibility in professional practice implies two components: a comprehensive knowledge of the relevant discipline and the appropriate skills to practice it. The first one is now probably impossible to achieve. There is evidence that the growth in scientific papers exceeds the number that are actually read. Extensive knowledge of the field is already necessary when obtaining an informed consent. There is a legal obligation to describe to the patient all possible diagnostic and therapeutic options. To fulfil this requirement every neurosurgeon should maintain up-dated knowledge of the current clinical developments. In practice explanation given to the patient is usually not extended to all newest technologies especially if their availability is limited or they are still under trial. Whether this is right and liable to suits has not been established [7].

It is generally accepted that up-to-date skills in new technologies can not be acquired by self teaching. Formal training with those who have already mastered the method is indispensable. Failure to fulfil this requirement may lead to legal consequences as in a case of incompetent performance of key-hole surgery [2, 5].

## Economy and Progress

Neurosurgeons to a greater extent than the majority of other specialists are affected by the changes in medical technologies, economic limitations in medicine and involvement of legal issues in the management of patients [10]. Those issues are relevant for the individuals, but they also influence the development of the speciality and its' future. Responsibility for the best possible management of the patients with neurosurgical diseases is a moral obligation of both: the individuals and of the professional societies. As a result of the rising costs of many new medical technologies it is not possible any more to maintain an old statement from the Hippocratic oath that every patient is given treatment regardless of its expense.

The Code of Ethics of the American Association of Neurological Surgeons in paragraph IIA obliges a neurosurgeon to provide the best patient care that available resources and circumstances can provide. Every patient has a right to be treated according to established standards, and regardless of the reasons for not providing such treatment there is legal responsibility for this failure. It is not clear who should be sued if this requirement is not met: a neurosurgeon, head of department, director of the hospital or minister of finance [9]. In some countries it is the state that holds the responsibility. Formally if a patient is treated inadequately as a result of general underinvestment in the health care system, there is still responsibility of the state for the situation. The courts base their judgement in such cases on common sense. It is obvious that even in the wealthiest countries there is no chance to offer everything to everyone. In judging individual claims it is considered what standard of treatment should be provided in a country with a defined economy, history and setting. The law is not precise in this respect which places a great responsibility on juries. Brain tumour diagnosis can serve as an example. CT is now a commonly accepted standard in the majority of countries. There may be sometimes local difficulties in obtaining this examination which can not be an excuse for a delay in the diagnosis and the court would consider the state responsible for failing to provide this standard examination. On the other hand claims that failure to execute some high-tech diagnosis like PET or treatment using boron neutron capture therapy would be rejected [9].

## Claims for Medical Negligence Related to new Technologies

There are legal suits associated with the use of new medical technologies. For example complaints against doctors performing minimal access surgery in the last decade rose steadily [5]. Those complaints usually resulted from inadequate training and experience, too great an expectation of the patients and enthusiasm of the surgeons for this new method leading to poorly justified extension of indications for its' use. The knowledge that is needed to practice contemporary neurosurgery goes far beyond the purely medical disciplines. Already now, but more so in the near future competence in medical information technology and data systems will be a commonplace professional skill.

Application of new achievements in medicine can have sometimes strange consequences. An interesting verdict has been given in 1980 by the court in the USA in case Curlender against Bioscience Laboratories USA. A child with Tay-Sachs genetic disorder was to be compensated by the Laboratories for being borne with the defect after imprecise genetic examination and counselling given to his parents.

This is known as right of non-existence. This verdict carries a risk of stigmatisation of those with genetic defects along the lines: look, he/she should not be borne. But people are different, nobody is genetically perfect. Beethoven had multiple genetic disorders, but mankind owes a lot to him. If this line of argument develops there will be a theoretical possibility for a child to sue the parents for genetic disorders. In order to reduce the financial risk related to investments and usage of new technologies institutions and individuals are requesting opinions on medical practice issues from Medical Associations and other institutions. AANS has carried on a Neurosurgical Clinical Procedure Review Program (NCPRP) in which a review of position papers related to clinical procedures previously evaluated by various technology, drug and procedures assessment committees. This served to recommend replacement of outmoded procedures by newer, better ones. This process involves evaluation of the scientific methods used previously in the evaluation of the procedure. In neurosurgery NCPRP evaluated among many others discography, facet rhizotomy and a variety of diagnostic procedures. This good intended activity has placed the committees at risk of legal liability. Suits were made for economic loss resulting from the opinions regarding a procedure as being not acceptable or providing no real benefits. The recommendations of the committees, even those very benign in nature can have a negative impact on reimbursement for the procedure. Those who invested in the new technology sue those unfavourable decisions referring among others to antitrust law [8]. As a result the Technology Assessment Committee was obliged to send all procedure reviews to persons known to hold a variety of views [8].

Development and introduction of new technologies in neurosurgery is certainly beneficial for the patients but there are numerous hazards in this process if the ethical rules are not strictly followed.

## References

1. Amdur RJ, Biddle C (1997) Institutional review board approval and publication of human research results. JAMA 277: 909–914
2. Anonymous (1995) Brit Med J 311: 213
3. Bolam v Friern HMC (1957) 2All ER 118
4. Garfield J (1992) Report of the activities and its results of the Ethico-Legal Committee of the EANS. Acta Neurochir (Wien) 116: 83–93
5. Goldwin H (1998) Minimal access surgery. Int J MDU 12: 5–7
6. Loew F (1992) Ethics in neurosurgery. Acta Neurochir (Wien) 116: 187–189
7. Peysner J (1996) Boiled frogs and distant sails. J Med Def Uni 10: 2–3
8. Ramsey L, Williams H, Tolchin S (1992) Clinical procedures review: another casualty of a litigious society. Surg Neurol 38: 173–178
9. Safian. M (1998) Prawo i medycyna. Ochrona praw jednostki a dylematy medycyny wspót czesnej. Instytut Wymiaru Spra-wiedliwości, Warszawa
10. Trojanowski T (1996) Medicolegal pitfalls in neurosurgical practice. Neuro Surg. In: Palmer JD (ed) Churchill Livingstone, New York, pp 28–31

Correspondence: Prof. Dr. Tomasz Trojanowski, Department of Neurosurgery and Paediatric Neurosurgery, University Medical School, Jaczewskiego 8, 20 950 Lublin, Poland.

Acta Neurochir (1999) [Suppl] 74: 89–92
© Springer-Verlag 1999

# Professional Integrity: On Moral Education in Medicine

**E. Schroten**

Center for Bio-ethics and Health Law University of Utrecht, Utrecht, The Netherlands

In his invitational letter Professor Van Alphen asked me to present a paper on 'How to teach our students and residents in moral behaviour?'. Thinking about the meaning of this question, I realized that it asks more than merely telling you something about teaching medical ethics in neurosurgery. Let me explain.

'Ethics' can be defined as: systematic moral reflection or, more precisely, systematic reflection about morals and morality. 'Morals' and 'morality' refer to moral behaviour, of individuals, groups, societies or cultures, i.e. behaviour seen from the perspective of right or wrong, good or bad, virtues, norms and values. And 'systematic reflection' means: a way of thinking and arguing which is rational and methodological, and open for discussion. Against this background it may be clear, then, that 'medical ethics' means: systematic reflection about morals and morality in medicine. Taken in this sense, medical ethics is a subject which can be taught.

But can moral behaviour be taught as well? And professional integrity? There is a classic question in ethics: Is virtue teachable? Virtues like integrity, and moral behaviour in general, refer to a deeper layer in human existence than our intellectual capacities. They refer to conviction, motivation, character, personality and will. In other words, moral behaviour is more than intellectual performance, more than reflection about morality. If virtue would be teachable, then knowing what ought to be done would imply doing it, which is not the case (as we all know).

In short: moral education is more (and more difficult!) than teaching ethics. I shall come back to this 'more' later on. Meanwhile, however, what I have said about the distinction between teaching ethics and teaching moral behaviour is not meant to deny that teaching ethics is an important part of moral educa-tion. Knowing what ought to be done may not imply doing it, it is, nevertheless, an important condition for it. Let us therefore pay attention to the question: How to teach ethics in medicine?

In medicine (neurological surgery) one cannot pre-suppose a philosophical training. Therefore, in my Centre, we prefer a bottom up approach. It means that we take our starting point not in ethical theory but in a case study, trying to develop an answer to the question what, in that specific case, ought to be done (and what not). In the course of such a case study (for instance withholding or withdrawing treatment in case of severe brain damage) you use as much ethical theory as you need for finding an answer. In the jargon of my disci-pline this way of doing ethics is called applied ethics.

Applied medical ethics can be seen as moral decision making in medicine. Taken in this sense, it is supposed to be more than a nice discussion on the moral aspects of a specific case, however interesting that may be. For moral decision making, at least (1) a pathway and (2) a framework are required.

(1) In the teaching programme of my Centre we use, as a pathway in applied ethics, a so called step-by-step-design, which runs as follows:

*Phase I: Explicity*

1. What is the moral question?
2. Which possibilities for action are open on first sight?
3. Which factual information is lacking?

*Phase II: Analysis*

4. Who are involved in this moral issue?
5. Which arguments are relevant for answering the moral question?

*Phase III: Weighing*

6. What is the importance of these arguments for this case?
7. Which possible action is preferable on the basis of weighing the arguments?

*Phase IV: Action*

8. Which concrete steps follow from it?

This design is, I hope, relatively clear by itself. It is important to keep in mind that it is used in case studies.

(2) The framework in which this design is used is the so-called reflective equilibrium model. Originally, this model stems from [5], who introduced it as a model for developing a general theory of justice. It has been adapted for other purposes by several scholars, in the context of our Centre [9]. In its adapted form it can be seen as a useful way of handling practical moral problems, meant as a coherence model, aiming at a reflective equilibrium of five aspects in moral reasoning, namely:

*Moral Judgments (or Intuitions)*

We all have moral judgments, intuitions or feelings about what ought (not) to be done in certain cases. In order to avoid moral bias and sheer subjectivism, these judgments should be clarified and brought into critical interaction with more general moral and non-moral considerations, such as:

*Moral Principles*

As many may know, in biomedical ethics four principles, play an important role in the doctor-patient-relationship [1]:

– (Respect for) autonomy (of the patient)
– Nonmalificence ( the classic *'primum non nocere'*)
– Beneficence
– Justice (i.e. *'iustitia distributiva'*).

In biomedical ethics, there is much debate on the relationship of these four principles. I cannot elaborate on this discussion here, but later on I want to make some remarks on the specification of these basic principles.

*( Morally Relevant) Facts*

Moral reasoning is associated with norms and values, and rightly so. However, in applied ethics (like biomedical ethics) relevant factual information, such as diagnosis and prognosis, is very important for moral reasoning. It means per implication that professional competence and skill is important as well. "The components of medical competence are clinical judgment, medical knowledge, clinical skills, humanistic attitudes, communication skills, and continuing education" [7].

*Background Theories*

Here one can think of the philosophy of medicine, culture and religion. In my country, part of Western Europe, although it is secularized, medical ethics is still influenced by Judaism, Christianity and Humanism. If I may summarize it in one slogan, it runs: *Salus aegroti suprema lex* (the most important law is the wellbeing of the patient). The content of this ideal, however, is not a preriquisite of Western medicine. It could be the basis of a global medical ethics.

*Methodological Norms*

Mostly, in moral reasoning, these 'norms' are not formulated explicitly. They are, rather, presupposed. Looking for a reflective equilibrium requires rational discourse, according to the laws of logic, in mutual respect for each others arguments. In other words, what Habermas calls a *'herrschaftsfreie Diskussion'*.

This Reflective Equilibrium Model is very useful in pluralistic societies and different cultural settings, for it does not favour a specific type of belief. It requires an attitude of openness and respect for each other's ideas and beliefs, aiming at a rational discourse concerning the tenability and relevance of them. Therefore, it may be a good model for the Eurasian Academy of Neurological Surgery, which is a pluralistic community of scholars.

However, as we saw already, moral education is more than teaching ethics. I promised to come back to this 'more'. Moral education in medicine aims at professional integrity. Let me try to point out some features which I think to be important in this context. By the way, some aspects from above may come in from another angle.

*Professional Competence and Skill*

To avoid misunderstanding, it may be adequate to underline that moral education in medicine means that professional competence is of secondary importance. On the contrary, I would say, moral behaviour in a professional context, such as neurosurgery, means that competence and skill are presupposed.

## Selection

Keeping this in mind, it is good to realize that selection of students and residents is important. Not only academic capacities, but also motivation, character, kindness and common sense are qualities to look at.

## Attitude

In this time of impressive developments in biomedical science and technology it is of great importance that surgeons are educated in being *physicians*, which means that an attitude of care and patient-orientedness is to be expected [8]. Although surgeons are mostly 'do-ers', critical reflection on what they are doing and on what is going on in their discipline, an awareness of what is called the technological imperative, as well as a sound form of self-criticism (which is not to be equated with hesitation!) should be part of their attitude.

## Professional Code

A professional code is not a loincloth or an alibi for sailing under false colours. It should set the moral boundaries, especially for what is not acceptable. It is good medical practice concentrated on a certain discipline, such as neurological surgery. A certain form of control and of dealing with complaints should be part of a professional code.

## Role of Tutor

In moral education the role of the tutor is of paramount importance. It is a very delicate one as well, because the tutor-pupil relationship is characterized by a tension between authority and autonomy, certainly in morality. I cannot elaborate here on the ethics of teaching ethics [6], but I would stress that the attitude and the example of the tutor in moral education is more influential than ethical textbooks. It may be good to point out here that, in the tutor-pupil relationship, authority has a place. Moral education is not to be reduced to a '*herrschaftsfreie Diskussion*' in ethics (as has been indicated in the context of the reflective equilibrium model). It may be clear, however, that authority in moral education is a very delicate topic. Let me put it (too) shortly: A tutor should prove to be worthy of authority!

## Teaching Ethics

It has been said already: In moral education teaching ethics is important. Therefore, it may be interesting to come back, as promised, to the issue of specifying the above mentioned four basic principles of biomedical ethics. As an example of such a specification I want to use a recent consensus document from the UK, on what should be the core curriculum for medical ethics and law. It has been published in the [4], with a summary in the [2]. It is, by the way, interesting to be aware of the fact that already in 1987 the British Medical Association (BMA) has called upon the General Medical Council (GMC) to instruct all medical schools to provide 'identifiable and substantial courses on medical ethics in their undergrate curricula' [3]. It may be seen as a sign that it is not easy to get moral education into the medical curricula, not only in the UK but everywhere.

In the consensus document, twelve issues are brought forward, which should be present in any medical curriculum.

- Informed consent and refusal of treatment (respect for patient autonomy).
- The clinical relationship: truthfulness, trust and good communication (virtues in clinical practice).
- Confidentiality (privacy and trust).
- Medical research (ethical and legal tensions in doing research on patients, human volunteers and animals).
- Human reproduction (status of the human embryo, prenatal screening, abortion).
- The new genetics (genetic screening and counselling, gene therapy, treating the abnormal vs. improving the normal).
- Children (children's rights, incompetence, moral & legal significance of age, proxy decision making).
- Mental disorders and disabilities (definitions, treatment without consent, conflicts of interests between patient, family and community.
- Life, death, dying and killing (duty of care, justifications for non-provision of life prolonging treatment, euthanasia, transplantation).
- Vulnerabilities created by the duties of doctors and medical students (public expectations, dealing with mistakes, complaints, whistle-blowing, involvement

in police work and torture (and, we could add, drugs in sport!).

– Resource allocation (equity and just distribution of scarce health resources).

– Rights (what rights are, importance of human rights for medical ethics).

This is a very good initiative, which should be supported where possible. I would underline that these topics should also be dealt with in professional codes in medicine, such as in neurosurgery. It goes without saying that an adaptation to the specific issues in neurological surgery is required. The only thing I would like to add to this list of topics is some training in the use of a pathway in ethical reasoning and some information about a moral framework, as I have indicated above.

Last but not least: *Organisation*

What I like in the above mentioned consensus statement in the UK is that it includes organisational requirements, such as full integration of medical ethics and law in the curriculum and a full-time senior academic staff member in ethics and law with relevant experience. Moral education in medicine is not a question of certain initiatives of good-willing individuals, but it must have a structural basis. In my view this should not only be implemented in the medical curriculum but in the context of the professional code as well. An adequate professional code requires an ethical committee which is not only charged to monitor what is going on in the profession, but also the developments

in science and technology in order to adjust, if necessary, the professionals code every five years.

Let me summarize my contribution by using the maxim of your Academy: '*Humanitati et arti*', for humanity and for skill. For an ethicist like me it is interesting to see that humanity comes first, and rightly so. But the word 'et' means that scientifically based skill is on the same level. Humanity and skill should go hand in hand. This, according to me, should be the ideal for moral education in neurological surgery.

## References

1. Beauchamp TL, Childress JF (1994) Principles of biomedical ethics, 4th edn. Oxford University Press New York Oxford
2. Bulletin of Medical Ethics (1998) 138: 3–4
3. Evans D (1987) Health care ethics: a pattern for learning. J Med Ethics 13: 127–131
4. J Med Ethics (1998) 24: 188–1992
5. Rawls J (1971) A theory of justice. Oxford University Press, London
6. Schroten E (1997) Die Ethik der Vermittlung von Ethik in der Medizin. In: Reiter-Theil S (Hrsg) Vermittlung Medizinischer Ethik. Theorie und Praxis in Europa. Nomos Verlagsgesellschaft, Baden-Baden, SS 44–50
7. Tew JM Jr (1984) Medical competence – education and ethics'. Neurosurgery 15: 1
8. Van Alphen H, August M (1990) Neurosurgery and medical ethics: considerations in the light of future developements. Prog Clin Neurosci 6: 1–7
9. Van Willigenburg T et al (1993), Ethiek in praktijk. Van Gorcum, Assen, pp 55ff

Correspondence: Egbert Schroten, Ph.D., Center for Bioethics and Health Law University of Utrecht, Heidelberglaan 2, 3584 CS Utrecht, The Netherlands.

Acta Neurochir (1999) [Suppl] 74: 93–96

# Ethical Requisites of Basic Knowledge, Diagnostic Procedures and Operative Techniques in Neurosurgical Training and Practice

**R. Van den Bergh**

University of Leuven, Leuven, Belgium

## Introduction

Since the time the pioneering days of neurosurgery have ended, a certain trivialization has occurred in this highly select discipline. The consequences are important: lessened professional pride, and diminished feeling of belonging to a special group, to an elite. This evolution is caused by the fast growing number of neurosurgeons and by certain aspects of democratization.

Nevertheless, neurosurgeons, neurologists and other neuroscientists belong to a special group, because the object of their knowledge and their care is primarily the Central Nervous System, the most characteristic and the most highly evolved organ of man, homo sapiens sapiens. The CNS, and more specifically the brain, is the seat of personality, intellect, affect, emotions and speech. All this means that ethics have a very special importance and significance in neurosurgical practice and even more in neurosurgical training.

I propose to consider the following requirements of ethics in the field of neurosurgery:

1. The necessity of acquiring a thorough basic knowledge, in the first place of topographical neuro-anatomy.
2. The art of diagnosing neurosurgical disorders.
3. The discipline of identifying the surgical indications, including the correct choice of the proper neurosurgical technique, and avoiding both interventionism and unfounded abstentionism.
4. The efficient and logical application of permanently evolving techniques and modern instruments, including the operation microscope, laser, ultrasound aspirator, stereotaxy and neuronavigation systems.

## Thorough Knowledge of Neuro-Anatomy

It is self-evident that the study of anatomy is a prerequisite for every branch of surgery. However, the anatomy of the CNS is exceedingly more complex and compact than that of other organs or systems. Studying in atlases and text books is insufficient for a candidate neurosurgeon. Dissection exercises of the human brain, including the three-dimensional fiber dissection technique after freezing, under the guidance of an experienced teacher, are indispensable.

During a brain operation the neurosurgeon has to keep in mind all the time the nearby localization of invisible but important brain structures. He has to know exactly the topography of hidden structures he is approaching.

Even more than the neural structures, the cerebral vasculature is grossly unknown to many young neurosurgeons. Blood vessels, arteries and veins, are "mal" treated without considering the consequences for brain structures at a certain distance. Neurosurgeons have to know to which vascular territory a certain brain area belongs, or which vessels provide for a certain brain structure. They have to know the course, position and branching modalities of the most important vessels. They must avoid the interruption of any vessel without important reason and without having identified the vessel.

## Adequate Diagnosis of Neurosurgical Disorders

The undervaluation and neglect of the clinical examination is a general phenomenon in recent years. The clinical examination, including history taking of patient and family, remains the base for an adequate diagnosis. In neurology and neurosurgery, this is even more important than in other branches of medicine. The art of clinical examination should be restored.

It is unethical to start initially a whole battery of technical investigations, including CT scan, MRI, EMG and angiography, a fortiori if some of them are invasive. These examinations are of course useful and the technological advances present new possibilities, but they have to be used in a purposeful manner. Moreover the neurosurgeon has to feel himself involved and has to be able to interpret the imaging studies taking into account the history of the complaints and viewing the results in the frame of the clinical context. All too often surgery is decided even when the clinical findings do not correlate with the radiological data.

The danger also exists that imaging abnormalities without pathological significance lead to unnecessary surgery. With the modern techniques all kinds of previously unrecognized or underestimated anomalies are regularly discovered (midline brain cysts, both supra- and infratentorial, temporal arachnoid cysts, small congenital and often stable tumours in the suprasellar region etc.). Obviously it is unethical to operate on these anomalies, when there is no correlation at all with the patient's complaints.

### Identification of the Correct Neurosurgical Indication

The correct indication for neurosurgery results from an adequate diagnosis of the disorder. Otherwise, once a surgical treatment is in principle decided on, the correct choice of the proper neurosurgical technique has to be made and is extremely important.

It is the ethical duty of a neurosurgeon to remain informed about the continuing evolution, allowing him to choose and to apply the ideal current technique for a given patient with a certain pathology. In the process he has to inform the patient precisely on the advantages and drawbacks of the technique, and its potential dangers, something which is also true for the pre-operative diagnostic investigations.

The neurosurgeon should know the limits of his own skill and competence, and also of the local possibilities concerning equipment and skilled medical and paramedical personnel. If it appears that he does not possess the necessary expertise with the specific technique, indicated in a certain patient, it is his ethical and moral duty to inform the patient and to refer him to another

member of his team who has more experience in that domain, or even to a colleague in an other hospital. In this situation, and especially concerning the patient's informed consent, it is recommended to note all discussions and decisions truthfully in the files. Finally, it has to be pointed out that the referring neurosurgeon should place the most complete information and all medical data at the disposal of his colleague who is performing the surgery.

When performing surgery in two hospitals, one must make sure that in the "second" center the technical equipment and facilities are sufficient, that postoperative care is possible in the best conditions, and that qualified personnel is available.

Lastly, I want to scrutinize interventionism and abstentionism (or minimalism). Interventionism is unethical. Immediately the dramatic rise in operations for so-called lumbar instability and "black disks" comes into mind. Other examples are operations for adult hydrocephalus in patients with Normal Pressure Hydrocephalus, without the typical clinical syndrome with the triad of mnestic dementia, gait apraxia and urinary incontinence, and/or without performing CSF pressure measurements.

Furthermore, the plethora of neurosurgeons in some countries has created a dangerous and unethical situation by inciting overconsumption, by diminishing the expertise in rarely performed and technically difficult operations, and by pushing neurosurgeons to perform operations beyond their competence and experience.

Because of these reasons, too small centers with a single neurosurgeon are not advisable. In a team, the members can supplement each others shortcomings, they can impart knowledge and surgical expertise, and critically protect each other from wrong decisions.

In this respect, the potential danger of the ever growing commercialization of medicine has to be mentioned briefly. The high investments for the acquisition of new technologies (e.g. neuronavigation) have to be paid for inciting the neurosurgeon to use these devices even in cases where they do not really apply. This places an unethical financial burden on the patient, his insurance company, or the whole society. Just as disputable from the ethical point of view is the practice of using certain devices (e.g. osteosynthesis screws, disk replacement cages, etc.) not because of any proven scientific value, but because of financial rewards from the manufacturing companies.

When one encounters severe incompetence or serious professional faults in a colleague, these should be pointed out to him/her in a correct and friendly way. When this has no results, the proper instances or the Board should be notified. When it becomes clear that a young person in training is not apt for neurosurgery, an other option should be advised as early as possible.

Abstentionism is sometimes an expression of prudence but it can also be unethical. Some neurosurgeons, insufficiently trained for difficult tumour surgery, or with insufficient ability, often consider the tumour as inoperable or limit themselves to a biopsy or a partial resection. They seem to trust overmuch in a biopsy, which they furthermore sometimes perform in a risky manner, because their anatomical insight is insufficient or because the stereotactical frame they have at their disposal, is not suited for certain localisations (e.g. low temporal or posterior fossa biopsies).

Many gliomas which appear to be high grade on stereotactic biopsy, can have a fair prognosis after a skillful resection that is as complete as possible, followed by radiotherapy. It is unethical not to give the patient all possible chances for a meaningful survival. When the neurosurgeon has a tendency to be conservative or minimalistic in these cases, because he either consciously or unconsciously estimates himself not adequate, he should refer the patient to an other member of his team with more experience in this kind of surgery.

In the fifties and sixties these tumours were operated on in an excellent fashion because the neurosurgeons of the pioneering days and the expansion era, small in numbers, mastered the whole spectrum of neurosurgery. The present plethora and the subspecialisation (functional and stereotactic neurosurgery, vascular neurosurgery, spinal neurosurgery, spinal cord neurosurgery, skull base neurosurgery, etc) has created excellent neurosurgeons, reaching very high standards in a limited domain, but less competent in other fields.

## The Efficient Application of Modern Instruments and Technologies

The use of novel instruments and modern technology is at present posing many ethical problems. When a well trained, experienced and skilled neurosurgeon uses modern techniques like operation microscope, laser, minimally invasive techniques and neuronavigation, this will represent for himself and for his patients an enrichment. It is however illusory to think that a less skilled neurosurgeon will be able to compensate for his shortcomings by using these techniques: he will not become better but more dangerous.

New instruments should be at the service of the neurosurgeon if his operations become safer or more efficient because of them. They must however not become a goal in themselves. The application of laser can be useful in certain tumour types with certain localizations and vascularisation patterns. However, when one wants to use the laser in tumours which can be removed simply and safely by classical techniques, laser may inflict more damage to the surrounding brain parenchyma and the peritumoural blood vessels than is necessary and ethically justifiable.

An even larger problem occurs with the so-called minimally invasive techniques. The number of real and logical indications in neurosurgery is very restricted, with the exception of lesions located in the ventricles and some cisterns. Using this technology with video camera and television screen for the removal of a classical herniated disc renders the operation unnecessarily long, complicated and dangerous. Small migrated disc fragments may escape the exploration, and a meticulous and secure haemostasis can be difficult.

Neuronavigation is posing a special problem. Actually a young neurosurgeon, before practising this technique, should gradually develop his personal subjective orientation and "neuronavigation" qualities. He has to do this by a thorough study of topographical neuro-anatomy, and by the practice of classical neurosurgical techniques for a sufficiently long period. Only then can he fruitfully apply stereotactic neuronavigation. He must be aware of the drawbacks and the relativity of navigation parameters (e.g. the changes in the anatomical relationships by brain shift due to loss of CSF or progressive tumour extirpation). The application of navigation technology by a neurosurgeon who does not thoroughly master neuro-anatomy is unethical and dangerous.

## Conclusions

1. Thorough knowledge of topographical neuro-anatomy based not only on the study of atlases and text books but also on practical brain dissection exercises, is a prerequisite in the neurosurgeon's training.
2. An adequate diagnosis of a neurosurgical disorder has to be founded in the first place on the clinical examination. Technical examinations have to be executed afterwards and in a purposeful manner.

The neurosurgeon has to study the imaging results himself in order to interpret them in the frame of the clinical context. It is unethical to operate on radiological or MRI findings without sufficient correlation with the clinical signs and symptoms.

3. It is the ethical duty of a neurosurgeon to apply the ideal current technique for a given patient. He should refer this patient to a colleague with more experience in that domain if he does not possess the necessary expertise.

   Interventionism and unfounded abstentionism are both unethical.

4. Novel instruments and new techniques should be used if a given operation becomes safer and more efficient because of them. It poses however an ethical problem if they become a goal in themselves.

## Acknowledgements

The author wishes to thank Frank Van Calenbergh, M.D., for fruitful discussions about these ethical issues and for assistance with the translation of the original dutch text.

Correspondence: Prof. Dr. R. Van den Bergh, Heidebergstraat 248a, 3010 Leuven, Belgium.

# Index

SpringerNeurology

Alexander Baethmann, Nikolaus Plesnila,
Florian Ringel, Jörg Eriskat (eds.)

Current Progress in the Understanding
of Secondary Brain Damage
from Trauma and Ischemia

1999. VIII, 119 pages. 28 partly coloured figures. Hardcover DM 120,–, öS 840,–
Reduced price for subscribers to "Acta Neurochirurgica" (–10 %)
DM 108,–, öS 756,– (All prices are recommended retail prices)
ISBN 3-211-83313-7. Acta Neurochirurgica, Supplement 73

Information is provided from the basic and clinical sciences on the mechanisms damaging the brain from trauma or ischemia. New aspects involve the endoplasmic reticulum, mitochondrial failure, pathobiology of axonal injury, molecular signals activating glial elements, or the emerging therapeutical role of neurotrophins. Experimental issues involve a better analysis of the ischemic penumbra, the salvagable tissue.

Therapeutic contributions reach from the environmental influence to gene expression, including neuroprotection, such as hibernation – mother nature's experiment – or hypothermia which is reported to induce cell swelling. Treatment issues deal also with thrombolysis and combination therapies, or with the clearance of adverse blood components – LDL/fibrinogen – by a novel procedure using heparin.

Other highlights are discussing the specificities of pediatric vs. adult brain trauma, or the evolving role of the Apolipoprotein-E e4 gene in severe head injury. An update is also provided on an online assessment of the patient management during the pre- and early hospital phase in Southern Bavaria.

The empirical observation of neuroworsening is analyzed in further details, whether this is a specificity autonomously driving the posttraumatic course. Finally, the unsolved question why drug trials in severe head injury have failed so far in view of the promising evidence from the laboratory is subjected to an expert analysis.

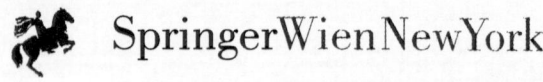

SpringerWienNewYork

Sachsenplatz 4–6, P.O.Box 89, A-1201 Wien, Fax +43-1-330 24 26, e-mail: books@springer.at, Internet: http://www.springer.at
New York, NY 10010, 175 Fifth Avenue • D-14197 Berlin, Heidelberger Platz 3 • Tokyo 113, 3–13, Hongo 3-chome, Bunkyo-ku

SpringerNeurology

Iver A. Langmoen, Tryggve Lundar,
Rune Aaslid, Hans-J. Reulen (eds.)

# Neurosurgical Management of Aneurysmal Subarachnoid Haemorrhage

1999. VII, 177 pages. 66 figures. Hardcover DM 140,–, öS 980,–
Reduced price for subscribers to "Acta Neurochirurgica" (–10 %)
DM 126,–, öS 882.– (All prices are recommended retail prices)
ISBN 3-211-83256-4. Acta Neurochirurgica, Supplement 72

The book presents state-of-the-art management of aneurysmal subarachnoid haemorrhage by a group of internationally highly recognized neurosurgeons. All aspects of neurosurgical diagnoses and treatment of aneurysmal subarachnoid haemorrhage are covered. There are separate chapters by world leading surgeons on transcranial doppler, treatment in intensive care unit, mechanisms, diagnoses and treatment of vasospasms, titanium aneurysm clips, surgical methods for treating aneurysms in the cavernous sinus, surgical methods for posterior circulation of aneurysms, surgical methods for anterior circulation aneurysms and methods for giant aneurysms, as well as long-term follow-up and neuro-psychological consequences.

## Contents

A Tribute to Helge Nornes • Intracranial Aneurysms and Subarachnoid Hemorrhage Management of the Poor Grade Patient • Etiology of Cerebral Vasospasm • Hemodynamics of Cerebrovascular Spasm • The Role of Transcranial Doppler in the Management of Patients with Subarachnoid Haemorrhage – a Review • Neurointensive Care of Aneurysmal SAH • Virtues and Drawbacks of Titanium Alloy Aneurysm Clips • A Combined Transorbital-Transclinoid and Transsylvian Approach to Carotid-Ophthalmic Aneurysms Without Retraction of the Brain • Extradural Approach to Intracavernous ICA Aneurysms • Surgical Treatment of Anterior Circulation Aneurysms • Posterior Circulation Aneurysms. Technical Strategies Based on Angiographic Anatomical Findings and the Results of 60 Recent Consecutive Cases • Surgical Strategies for Giant Intracranial Aneurysms • Functional Outcome After Aneurysmal Subarachnoid Hemorrhage

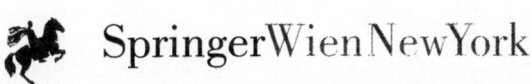

SpringerWienNewYork

Sachsenplatz 4–6, P.O.Box 89, A-1201 Wien, Fax +43-1-330 24 26, e-mail: books@springer.at, **Internet: http://www.springer.at**
New York, NY 10010, 175 Fifth Avenue • D-14197 Berlin, Heidelberger Platz 3 • Tokyo 113, 3–13, Hongo 3-chome, Bunkyo-ku